UNDERGROUND CLINICAL VIGNETTES

....

PATHOPHYSIOLOGY VOL. III

Classic Clinical Cases for
USMLE Step 1 Review [109 cases, 1st ed]

VIKAS BHUSHAN, MD
University of California, San Francisco, Class of 1991
Series Editor, Diagnostic Radiologist

CHIRAG AMIN, MD
University of Miami, Class of 1996
Orlando Regional Medical Center, Resident in Orthopaedic Surgery

TAO LE, MD
University of California, San Francisco, Class of 1996
Yale-New Haven Hospital, Resident in Internal Medicine

HOANG NGUYEN
Northwestern University, Class of 2000

ASHRAF ZAMAN, MBBS
New Delhi, India

©1999 by S2S Medical Publishing

Distributed by Blackwell Science, Inc.
Editorial Office:
Commerce Place, 350 Main Street, Malden, Massachusetts 02148, USA

Distributors
USA

Blackwell Science, Inc.
Commerce Place
350 Main Street
Malden, Massachusetts 02148
(Telephone orders: 800-215-1000 or
781-388-8250;
fax orders: 781-388-8270)

Canada

Login Brothers Book Company
324 Saulteaux Crescent
Winnipeg, Manitoba, R3J 3T2
(Telephone orders: 204-224-4068;
Telephone: 800-665-1148; fax: 800-665-0103)

Australia

Blackwell Science Pty, Ltd.
54 University Street
Carlton, Victoria 3053
(Telephone orders: 03-9347-0300;
fax orders: 03-9349-3016)

Outside North America and Australia

Blackwell Science, Ltd.
c/o Marston Book Services, Ltd.
P.O. Box 269
Abingdon
Oxon OX14 4YN
England
(Telephone orders: 44-01235-465500;
fax orders: 44-01235-465555)

ISBN: 1-890061-32-8

Editor: Andrea Fellows
Typesetter: Vikas Bhushan using MS Word97
Printed and bound by Capital City Press

Printed in the United States of America
99 00 01 02 6 5 4 3

Contributors

....

RICHA VARMA
Cambridge Overseas Medical Training Programme, Class of 2001

SONAL SHAH
Ross University, Class of 2000

VIPAL SONI
UCLA School of Medicine, Class of 1999

Acknowledgments

. . . .

Throughout the production of this book, we have had the support of many friends and colleagues. Special thanks to our business manager, Gianni Le Nguyen. For expert computer support, Tarun Mathur and Alex Grimm. For design suggestions, Sonia Santos and Elizabeth Sanders.

For editing, proofreading, and assistance across the vignette series, we collectively thank Carolyn Alexander, Henry E. Aryan, Natalie Barteneva, Sanjay Bindra, Julianne Brown, Hebert Chen, Arnold Chin, Yoon Cho, Karekin R. Cunningham, A. Sean Dalley, Sunit Das, Ryan Armando Dave, Robert DeMello, David Donson, Alea Eusebio, Priscilla A. Frase, Anil Gehi, Parul Goyal, Alex Grimm, Tim Jackson, Sundar Jayaraman, Aarchan Joshi, Rajni K. Jutla, Faiyaz Kapadi, Aaron S. Kesselheim, Sana Khan, Andrew Pin-wei Ko, Warren S. Krackov, Benjamin H.S. Lau, Scott Lee, Warren Levinson, Eric Ley, Ken Lin, Samir Mehta, Gil Melmed, Joe Messina, Vivek Nandkarni, Deanna Nobleza, Darin T. Okuda, Adam L. Palance, Sonny Patel, Ricardo Pietrobon, Riva L. Rahl, Aashita Randeria, Marilou Reyes, Diego Ruiz, Anthony Russell, Sanjay Sahgal, Sonal Shah, John Stulak, Lillian Su, Julie Sundaram, Rita Suri, Richa Varma, Amy Williams, Ashraf Zaman and David Zipf. Please let us know if your name has been missed or mispelled and we will be happy to make the change in the next edition.

Table of Contents

· ·

CASE	SUBSPECIALTY	NAME
40	Heme/Onc	Eosinophilic Granuloma
41	Heme/Onc	Glucose-6-Phosphate Dehydrogenase
42	Heme/Onc	Hemochromatosis
43	Heme/Onc	Sickle Cell Anemia
44	Heme/Onc	Transfusion Reaction
45	Neurology	Alzheimer's Disease
46	Neurology	Benign Positional Vertigo
47	Neurology	Broca's Aphasia
48	Neurology	C1 Spinal Cord Injury
49	Neurology	Cauda Equina Syndrome
50	Neurology	Hemiballismus
51	Neurology	Hepatic Encephalopathy and Cirrhosis
52	Neurology	Huntington's Chorea
53	Neurology	Internuclear Ophthalmoplegia
54	Neurology	Klüver–Bucy Syndrome
55	Neurology	Mass in Jugular Foramen
56	Neurology	Meningioma
57	Neurology	Migraine
58	Neurology	Neuroblastoma
59	Neurology	Normal Pressure Hydrocephalus
60	Neurology	Pseudobulbar Palsy
61	Neurology	Wernicke's Encephalopathy
62	OB/Gyn	Dysmenorrhea
63	OB/Gyn	Fibrocystic Disease of the Breast
64	OB/Gyn	Gynecomastia with Testicular
65	OB/Gyn	Infiltrating Ductal Carcinoma
66	OB/Gyn	Inflammatory Carcinoma of Breast
67	OB/Gyn	Lobular Carcinoma of the Breast
68	OB/Gyn	Ovarian Teratoma
69	OB/Gyn	Polycystic Ovary Disease
70	OB/Gyn	Postpartum Hemorrhage
71	OB/Gyn	Vulvar Carcinoma
72	Ophthalmology	Presbyopia
73	Ophthalmology	Pseudotumor Cerebri
74	Ophthalmology	Retinitis Pigmentosa
75	Orthopedics	Anterior Cruciate Ligament Injury
76	Orthopedics	Avascular Necrosis of the Femoral Head
77	Orthopedics	Carpal Tunnel Syndrome
78	Orthopedics	Cervical Spondylosis
79	Orthopedics	Ewing's Sarcoma
80	Orthopedics	Herniated Disc
81	Orthopedics	Monteggia's Fracture
82	Orthopedics	Osteitis Fibrosa Cystica
83	Orthopedics	Scaphoid Fracture
84	Orthopedics	Shoulder Dislocation
85	Orthopedics	Slipped Capital Femoral Epiphysis
86	Otolaryngology	Cribriform Plate Fracture
87	Otolaryngology	Labyrinthitis

CASE	SUBSPECIALTY	NAME
88	Otolaryngology	Menière's Disease
89	Otolaryngology	Presbycusis
90	Otolaryngology	Sensorineural Hearing Loss with Neuroma
91	Pulmonology	Chronic Pulmonary Emphysema
92	Pulmonology	Hypersensitivity Pneumonitis
93	Pulmonology	Idiopathic Pulmonary Fibrosis (IPF)
94	Pulmonology	Sarcoidosis
95	Pulmonology	Tension Pneumothorax
96	Rheumatology	Gout
97	Rheumatology	Letterer–Siwe Disease
98	Rheumatology	Osteoarthritis
99	Rheumatology	Osteopetrosis
100	Rheumatology	Osteoporosis
101	Rheumatology	Polymyalgia Rheumatica
102	Rheumatology	Pseudogout
103	Rheumatology	Raynaud's Disease
104	Rheumatology	Septic Arthritis
105	Urology	Bladder Outlet Obstruction, Nephropathy
106	Urology	Hypertensive Renal Disease
107	Urology	Lupus Nephritis
108	Urology	Testicular Dysgenesis
109	Urology	Urate Nephropathy

Preface

. . . .

This series was developed to address the increasing number of clinical vignette questions on the USMLE Step 1. It is designed to supplement and complement *First Aid for the USMLE Step 1* (Appleton & Lange). Bi-directional cross-linking to appropriate High Yield Facts in the 1999 edition has been implemented

Each book uses a series of approximately 100 "**supra-prototypical**" **cases as a way to condense testable facts and associations.** The clinical vignettes in this series are designed to incorporate as many testable facts as possible into a cohesive and memorable clinical picture. The vignettes represent composites drawn from general and specialty textbooks, reference books, thousands of USMLE style questions and the personal experience of the authors and reviewers.

Although each case tends to present all the signs, symptoms, and diagnostic findings for a particular illness, **patients generally will not present with such a "complete" picture either clinically or on the Step 1 exam.** Cases are not meant to simulate a potential real patient or an exam vignette. All the **boldfaced "buzzwords" are for learning purposes** and are not necessarily expected to be found in any one patient with the disease.

Definitions of selected important terms are placed within the vignettes in (= SMALL CAPS) in parentheses. Other parenthetical remarks often refer to the pathophysiology or mechanism of disease. The format should also help students learn to present cases succinctly during oral "bullet" presentations on clinical rotations. The cases are meant to be read as a condensed review, not as a primary reference.

The information provided in this book has been prepared with a great deal of thought and careful research. This book should not, however, be considered as your sole source of information.

We invite your corrections and suggestions for the next edition of this book. For the first submission of each factual correction or new vignette, you will receive a personal acknowledgement and a free copy of the revised book. We prefer that you submit corrections or suggestions via electronic mail to vbhushan@aol.com. Please include "Underground Vignettes" as the subject of your message. If you do not have access to e-mail, use the following mailing address: S2S Medical Publishing, 1015 Gayley Ave, Box 1113, Los Angeles, CA 90024 USA.

Abbreviations

ABGs – arterial blood gases
ACA – anticardiolipin antibody
ACE – angiotensin-converting enzyme
ACTH – adrenocorticotropic hormone
ALT – alanine transaminase
Angio – angiography
AP – anteroposterior
APH – antepartum hemorrhage
ASO – anti-streptolysin O
AST – aspartate transaminase
AV - arteriovenous
BE – barium enema
BUN – blood urea nitrogen
CBC – complete blood count
CCU – coronary care unit
CMV – cytomegalovirus
CN – cranial nerve
CNS – central nervous system
COPD – chronic obstructive pulmonary disease
CAD – coronary artery disease
CSF – cerebrospinal fluid
CSOM – chronic suppurative otitis media
CT – computerized tomography
CXR – chest x-ray
DIC – disseminated intravascular coagulation
ECG – electrocardiography
Echo - echocardiography
EEG – electroencephalography
EGD – esophagogastroduodenoscopy
EM – electron microscopy
EMG – electromyography
ERCP – endoscopic retrograde cholangiopancreatography
ESR – erythrocyte sedimentation rate
FEV – forced expiratory volume
FNA – fine needle aspiration
FSH – follicle-stimulating hormone
FTA-ABS – fluorescent treponemal antibody absorption
FVC – forced vital capacity
G6PD – glucose-6-phosphate deficiency
GGF – gamma-glutamyl-transferase
GI – gastrointestinal
Hb – hemoglobin
hCG – human chorionic gonadotropin
HDL – high-density lipoprotein
HGPRT – hypoxanthine-guanine phosphoribosyltransferase
HIDA – hepato-iminodiacetic acid [scan]
HMA – homovanillic acid
HPI – history of present illness
HR – heart rate

Abbreviations - continued

. . . .

ID/CC – identification and chief complaint
Ig - immunoglobulin
IPF – idiopathic pulmonary fibrosis
IVC – inferior vena cava
IVP – intravenous pyelography
JVP – jugular venous pressure
KOH – potassium hydroxide
KUB – kidneys/ureter/bladder
LFTs – liver function tests
LH – luteinizing hormone
LP – lumbar puncture
Lytes – electrolytes
Mammo – mammography
MEN – multiple endocrine neoplasia
MR – magnetic resonance [imaging]
NSAID – nonsteroidal anti-inflammatory drug
Nuc – nuclear medicine
PA - posteroanterior
PAN – polyarteritis nodosa
PBC – primary biliary cirrhosis
PBS – peripheral blood smear
PCOS – polycystic ovarian syndrome
PCT – porphyria cutanea tarda
PE – physical exam
PET – positron emission tomography
PFTs – pulmonary function tests
PPH – postpartum hemorrhage
PTH – parathyroid hormone
PT – prothrombin time
PTT – partial thromboplastin time
SBFT – small bowel follow-through [barium study]
SISI – short-increment sensitivity index
SLE – systemic lupus erythematosus
TGI – thyroid growth immunoglobulin
THAA – tetrahydroaminoacridine
TIA – transient ischemic attack
TIBC – total iron-binding capacity
TSH – thyroid-stimulating hormone
TSI – thyroid-stimulating immunoglobulin
UA – urinalysis
UGI – upper GI [barium study]
US – ultrasound
V/Q – ventilation perfusion
VIN – vulvar intraepithelial neoplasia
VLDL – very low density lipoprotein
VMA – vanillylmandelic acid
VS – vital signs
VSD – ventricular septal defect
XR – x-ray

ID/CC	A 50-year-old woman is seen with complaints of recurrent, transient losses of consciousness (= SYNCOPE) and dizziness.
HPI	For the past few months she has had continuous mild to moderate fever, fatigue, sweating, and joint pains (= ARTHRALGIAS) and has experienced unexplainable breathlessness at rest (episodic pulmonary edema) that is relieved in a supine position and exacerbated by standing. She also complains of significant weight loss over the past year.
PE	VS: mild fever. PE: pallor and clubbing; on auscultation, S1 delayed and decreased in intensity and characteristic low-pitched sound (tumor plop) during early diastole, followed by a rumble; auscultatory findings varied with body position.
Labs	CBC: normochromic, normocytic anemia. Elevated ESR; increased IgG; blood cultures sterile. ECG: sinus rhythm.
Imaging	Echo (2D): characteristic echo-producing mass in left atrium. MR-Cardiac: globular mass in left atrium.
Gross Pathology	Single globular left atrial mass about 6 cm in diameter; pedunculated with fibrovascular stalk seen arising from interatrial septum in vicinity of fossa ovalis (favored site of atrial origin).
Micro Pathology	Stellate, multipotential mesenchymal myxoma cells mixed with endothelial cells; mature and immature smooth muscle cells and macrophages, all in an acid mucopolysaccharide matrix.
Treatment	Surgical excision utilizing cardiopulmonary bypass is curative.
Discussion	Myxomas are the most common type of primary cardiac tumors and may be located in any of the four chambers or rarely the valves. They are predominantly atrial with a 4:1 left-to-right ratio and are usually single. Although myxomas are benign, they can embolize, resulting in metastatic disease. Although the majority of myxomas are sporadic, some are familial with autosomal-dominant transmission; thus, echocardiographic screening of first-degree relatives is appropriate. **FIRST AID** p.246

ATRIAL MYXOMA

ID/CC	A 50-year-old male who was admitted to the CCU **three days ago** following an **MI** presents with **hypotension.**
HPI	The patient was thrombolyzed post-MI and was recovering well. He also complained of a mild fever but no chills or rigors.
PE	VS: tachycardia; weak, thready pulse; tachypnea; **hypotension.** PE: pallor; cool, moist skin; mild cyanosis of lips and digits; > 10-mmHg fall in arterial pressure with inspiration (= PULSUS PARADOXUS); **heart sounds muffled and JVP elevated; rise in level of venous pressure with inspiration** (= KUSSMAUL'S SIGN); lungs clear bilaterally.
Labs	Elevated cardiac enzymes (CK-MB, Troponin) as a result of recent acute MI.
Imaging	Echo: diastolic collapse of the right ventricle.
Gross Pathology	Rupture of the left ventricular wall with hemopericardium.
Micro Pathology	Ischemic coagulative necrosis of the affected myocardium, consisting of multiple erythrocytes and dead, anucleated myocytes.
Treatment	Emergency pericardiocentesis; treat shock by infusing fluid and isoproterenol; surgical repair of cardiac rupture subsequent to stabilization.
Discussion	Cardiac rupture most typically develops 3–10 days after the initial onset of the infarction, secondary to rupture of necrotic cardiac muscle; there is usually little warning before the sudden collapse, which is associated with acute cardiac tamponade and electromechanical dissociation. Papillary muscle rupture may also occur following an acute MI, resulting in mitral regurgitation and left ventricular failure.

CARDIAC TAMPONADE

ID/CC	A 35-year-old female **Asian** immigrant complains of weakness, **shortness of breath on exertion, and swelling of both feet.**
HPI	She also complains of **progressive abdominal distention** and fatigue. She was treated for **pulmonary tuberculosis** a few years ago.
PE	VS: mild hypotension; **small pulse pressure.** PE: peripheral cyanosis and cold extremities; pallor; neck veins distended; **JVP increases during inspiration** (= KUSSMAUL'S SIGN); pedal edema; moderate hepatomegaly, splenomegaly, and ascites; **reduced-intensity apical impulse, distant heart sounds, and early third heart sound (pericardial knock);** no pulsus paradoxus; no murmur or rub heard.
Labs	ECG: **low-voltage** QRS complexes with flattening of T wave (nonspecific); P-mitrale (in chronic cases). LFTs mildly abnormal (due to hepatic congestion); ascitic fluid **transudative** (low protein, high sugar). UA: proteinuria, no casts.
Imaging	CXR: **fibrosis** (old healed tuberculosis); heart shadow shows signs of **pericardial calcification.** Echo: **pericardial thickening.** CT: pericardial **calcification** and **thickening.**
Gross Pathology	Thick, dense, **fibrous obliteration of pericardial space with calcification** encasing the heart and **limiting diastolic filling.**
Micro Pathology	N/A
Treatment	**Complete pericardial resection** is the only definitive treatment; **antituberculous therapy** instituted when appropriate; diuretics; digitalis in presence of atrial fibrillation.
Discussion	**Tuberculosis** is the most common cause worldwide. Most cases now seen in the United States are idiopathic, but cases resulting from exposure to **radiation,** trauma, cardiac surgery, rheumatoid arthritis, or uremia have become more common. **FIRST AID** p.247

CONSTRICTIVE PERICARDITIS

ID/CC   A 23-year-old woman is seen with complaints of **excessive breathlessness, palpitations, fatigue, blood-streaked sputum** (= MILD HEMOPTYSIS), **and swelling of the feet** (= EDEMA).

HPI   She was diagnosed with **ventricular septal defect** (VSD) at birth, but her parents had refused surgery.

PE   VS: HR, BP normal; mild tachypnea; no fever. PE: **central cyanosis**; clubbing; JVP normal; left parasternal heave; P2 palpable; single second heart sound, predominantly loud P2 (due to pulmonary hypertension); pansystolic murmur along left sternal edge; ejection systolic murmur in pulmonary area; **mid-diastolic murmur** (= GRAHAM STEELL MURMUR OF PULMONARY REGURGITATION) **in pulmonary area that increased with inspiration** (= CARVALLO'S SIGN, INDICATING RIGHT-SIDED MURMUR).

Labs   ABGs: hypercapnia, hypoxia, and partly compensated respiratory acidosis. **Polycythemia.** ECG: **right ventricular hypertrophy** with right axis deviation; cardiac catheterization: right-to-left shunt, **pulmonary arterial hypertension**, and pulmonary regurgitation.

Imaging   Echo (with doppler): **VSD with right-to-left systolic shunt**; right ventricular enlargement and hypertrophy. CXR: pulmonary oligemia ("peripheral pruning") and greatly enlarged hilar pulmonary artery shadows; enlarged heart size.

Gross Pathology   N/A

Micro Pathology   N/A

Treatment   Heart-lung transplantation; surgical correction of a VSD is ideally performed before irreversible pulmonary vascular changes set in.

Discussion   The term "Eisenmenger's syndrome" applies to those defects in which **pulmonary vascular disease causes right-to-left shunt of blood**; Eisenmenger's complex is right-to-left shunt due to a large VSD.

. . . .

EISENMENGER'S COMPLEX

ID/CC	The case of a 50-year-old man who died of bleeding complications is discussed at an autopsy meeting owing to **peculiar vegetations seen on his mitral valve.**
HPI	He underwent surgery for **adenocarcinoma of the stomach.** Shortly before his death he was diagnosed as having **disseminated intravascular coagulation (DIC);** he subsequently died of bleeding complications.
PE	N/A
Labs	N/A
Imaging	N/A
Gross Pathology	Small (1- to 5-mm) **friable, sterile vegetations** loosely adherent to **mitral valve leaflets along lines of closure.**
Micro Pathology	Vegetations found to be **sterile fibrin and platelet thrombi** loosely attached **without evidence of inflammation** (bland) or valve damage.
Treatment	N/A
Discussion	Nonbacterial thrombotic endocarditis characteristically occurs in settings of **prolonged debilitating diseases** (e.g., cancer, particularly visceral adenocarcinomas) attributed to DIC, renal failure, chronic sepsis, or other malignancy-related **hypercoagulable states.** **FIRST AID** p.247

· ·

MARANTIC (NONBACTERIAL) ENDOCARDITIS

ID/CC	An 18-year-old white **male** complains of gradually progressing **shortness of breath** and **ankle swelling.**
HPI	His symptoms started following a **URI.** He also complains of **excessive fatigue and frequent chest pain.** He has no history of joint pains, skin rash, or involuntary movements (vs. rheumatic fever) and is neither hypertensive nor diabetic.
PE	VS: tachycardia; hypotension; no fever. PE: **elevated JVP;** pitting pedal edema; fine inspiratory rales at both lung bases; mild tender hepatomegaly, splenomegaly; **right-side S3;** murmurs of mitral regurgitation.
Labs	ASO titers not raised. CBC: lymphocytosis. Elevated ESR. ECG: **first-degree AV block with nonspecific ST-T** changes. **Coxsackievirus** isolated on pharyngeal washings; increased titers of serum antibodies to coxsackievirus; **elevated cardiac enzymes.**
Imaging	CXR: cardiomegaly and pulmonary edema. Echo: suggestive of dilated cardiomyopathy with low ejection fraction.
Gross Pathology	Flabby, dilated heart with foci of epicardial, myocardial, and endocardial petechial hemorrhages.
Micro Pathology	Endomyocardial biopsy: **diffuse infiltration by mononuclear cells, predominantly lymphocytes;** focal myofiber necrosis; focal fibrosis.
Treatment	Rest; control of congestive cardiac failure by diuretics, digitalis and vasodilators; cardiac transplant in intractable cases.
Discussion	Etiology is usually **coxsackie B** or other viruses; less often implicated are bacteria or fungi, *Trypanosoma cruzi* (Chagas' disease), hypersensitivity disease (SLE, drug reaction), radiation, and sarcoidosis. Diphtheria toxin also causes myocarditis by inhibiting eukaryotic elongation factor 2 (EF-2), thus inhibiting myocyte protein synthesis. May also be idiopathic. Young males are primarily affected.

MYOCARDITIS

ID/CC	A 50-year-old female who was admitted to the hospital for treatment of staphylococcal endocarditis complains of **severe pain at the site of antibiotic infusion.**
HPI	She was receiving **cloxacillin** (has propensity to cause thrombophlebitis) in addition to penicillin and gentamycin.
PE	Markedly **tender, cordlike inflamed area** found at site of infusion.
Labs	N/A
Imaging	Doppler venous ultrasound shows decreased venous compliance.
Gross Pathology	Intraluminal venous thrombus adherent to the vessel wall.
Micro Pathology	Acute inflammatory cells with endothelial wall damage and intraluminal thrombosis.
Treatment	Change infusion site frequently; NSAIDs; gentle support by means of a supporting bandage.
Discussion	Superficial thrombophlebitis most commonly occurs in **varicose veins** or in **veins cannulated for an infusion.** Spontaneous thrombophlebitis may occur in conditions such as polycythemia, polyarteritis nodosa, and Buerger's disease and as a sign of visceral cancer (thrombophlebitis migrans– Trousseau's sign).

THROMBOPHLEBITIS

ID/CC	A 15-year-old boy is referred to a cardiologist by a primary care physician for an evaluation of **recurrent dizzy spells.**
HPI	During his episodes he feels **intense anxiety with palpitations and breathlessness.** He has no history of chest pain or syncope and is normal in between episodes of dizziness.
PE	General and systemic physical exam normal; cardiac exam normal; otologic causes ruled out.
Labs	ECG: **short PR interval, wide QRS complex, and a slurred upstroke (= "DELTA WAVE") of QRS complex; R wave in V1 positive.** Electrophysiologic studies confirm **presence of a bypass tract** and its potential for development of life-threatening arrhythmia.
Imaging	N/A
Gross Pathology	N/A
Micro Pathology	N/A
Treatment	**Catheter radiofrequency ablation** of the accessory tract. Medical therapy (eg. Digoxin, verapamil, propranolol) is **not effective** in the presence of an accessory pathway.
Discussion	Wolff–Parkinson–White (WPW) syndrome is a term applied to patients with both preexcitation on ECG and paroxysmal tachycardia; in this case, the spells of dizziness could have been either paroxysmal supraventricular tachycardia or atrial fibrillation. An atrial premature contraction or a ventricular premature contraction generally initiates the reentrant tachycardia where the accessory tract usually conducts in a retrograde manner; the danger of atrial fibrillation lies in the fact that the accessory pathway may be capable of conducting very fast atrial rates, leading to a fast ventricular response that may degenerate into ventricular arrhythmias.

. . . .

WOLFF–PARKINSON–WHITE SYNDROME TYPE A

ID/CC	An 8-year-old boy presents with **intense pruritus and fluid-filled blisters** over his arms and legs.
HPI	He recently went on a camping trip with his classmates, during which he played the whole day in the bushes around the camping site.
PE	Typical **linear streaked vesicles over both arms and legs;** weepy and encrusted areas; numerous scratch marks over skin.
Labs	Gram stain and culture to rule out secondary infection; KOH preparation negative.
Imaging	N/A
Gross Pathology	Skin erythema and edema, with linear streaked vesicles.
Micro Pathology	Superficial perivascular **lymphocytic infiltration** around the blood vessels associated with edema of the dermal papillae and mast cell degranulation.
Treatment	Systemic and oral steroids.
Discussion	While at the campground the boy probably encountered poison ivy, a plant that produces low-molecular-weight oils (= URUSHIOLS) that induce contact hypersensitivity, which is a **cell-mediated, type IV hypersensitivity reaction.** The antigen is presented by the Langerhans cells to the helper lymphocytes. Both cell types travel to regional lymph nodes, where the antigen presentation is increased. Upon antigen challenge, the sensitized T-cells infiltrate the dermis and begin the immune response.

CONTACT DERMATITIS

ID/CC	A 35-year-old **man** presents with an **intensely pruritic rash** on his **elbows, knees, and back.**
HPI	He has **celiac sprue** and observes prescribed dietary precautions.
PE	PE: **bilaterally symmetrical** polymorphic skin lesions in the form of **small, tense vesicles on erythematous skin** (often in herpetiform groups); bullae and groups of pruritic papules over scapular and sacral areas, knees and elbows, and other **extensor surfaces.**
Labs	HLA-B8/DR w3 haplotype (particularly prone).
Imaging	N/A
Gross Pathology	**Polymorphous erythematous lesions,** including **papules, small vesicles, and larger bullae.**
Micro Pathology	Skin biopsy reveals characteristic **subepidermal blisters,** necrosis, and dermal papillary microabscesses; direct immunofluorescence studies reveal **granular deposits of IgA at tips of dermal papillae.**
Treatment	**Dapsone therapy** after confirming adequate glucose-6-phosphate dehydrogenase (G6PD) levels (dapsone produces hemolysis in G6PD-deficient individuals).
Discussion	A vesicular and extremely pruritic skin disease **associated with gluten sensitivity enteropathy** and IgA immune complexes deposited in dermal papillae; individuals with HLA-B8/DR-w3 haplotype are predisposed to developing the disease. **Males** are often more commonly affected, and peak incidence is in third and fourth decades. Patients on long-term dapsone therapy should be monitored for hemolysis and methemoglobinemia.

. . . .

DERMATITIS HERPETIFORMIS

ID/CC	A **16-year-old female** complains of **multiple nevi** on her skin.
HPI	She is concerned because an **aunt** who had a **similar illness** developed **malignant melanoma** and died of metastatic complications.
PE	**Multiple nevi measuring 6–15 mm** noted; nevi are variegated shades of pink, tan, and brown and seen on back, chest, buttocks, scalp, and breasts; **borders are irregular** and **poorly defined** but lack the scalloping of malignant melanoma; no regional lymphadenopathy noted.
Labs	N/A
Imaging	N/A
Gross Pathology	N/A
Micro Pathology	Skin biopsy reveals **cytologic and architectural atypia** with enlarged and fused epidermal nevus cell nests, **lentiginous hyperplasia**, and **pigment incontinence.**
Treatment	Sun protection; regular skin exam to detect development of malignant melanoma and biopsy of suspicious lesions.
Discussion	Dysplastic nevi are found in individuals with an autosomal-dominant predisposition to develop acquired nevi; these **may develop into malignant melanoma.**

. . . .

DYSPLASTIC NEVUS SYNDROME

ID/CC A 15-year-old male presents with fever of three days' duration, headache, **fleeting joint pains,** and a **reddish rash on the trunk** and left arm of two weeks' duration.

HPI N/A

PE VS: fever. PE: regional lymphadenopathy (axillary lymph nodes enlarged); mild neck stiffness; neurologic exam normal; **large (6- to 8-cm), annular, erythematous lesions with central blanching seen over left arm and trunk** (= ERYTHEMA CHRONICUM MIGRANS); no enanthema.

Labs ASO titer normal; IgM ELISA for *Borrelia burgdorferi* positive. ECG: normal. LP: CSF shows lymphocytic pleocytosis and increased proteins. *Borrelia* grown on Noguchi medium; specific intrathecal antibody to *Borrelia* demonstrated; joint fluid exam normal.

Imaging N/A

Gross Pathology N/A

Micro Pathology *Borrelia* demonstrable in skin lesions.

Treatment Amoxicillin.

Discussion Lyme disease is a tick-borne (*Ixodes* tick) illness caused by the spirochete *Borrelia burgdorferi*. Tick reservoirs include deer and mice. Lyme disease is divided into early disease (stages 1 and 2) and late disease (stage 3); **stage 1** is characterized by the presence of a distinctive skin lesion termed **erythema migrans** (EM, or erythema chronicum migrans). **Stage 2** is a disseminated phase of infection with manifestations in the **skin, CNS, musculoskeletal system, and heart.** Late disease, or **stage 3,** reflects persistent infection that is clinically manifest more than one year after the onset of disease. This stage most often involves the **skin, joints, and CNS.**

· ·

ERYTHEMA MIGRANS

ID/CC	A 4-year-old Japanese male presents with **fever and an extensive skin rash.**
HPI	A primary care physician had previously found the patient to have cervical adenitis; antibiotics were administered but achieved no response.
PE	VS: fever. PE: **conjunctival congestion;** dry, red lips; **erythematous palms and soles;** indurative edema of peripheral extremities; **desquamation of fingertips;** various rashes of trunk; **cervical lymphadenopathy** > 1.5 cm.
Labs	**Throat swab and culture sterile.** CBC: routine blood counts normal; further differential blood counts reveal increased B-cell activation and T-helper-cell lymphocytopenia. Paul–Bunnell test for infectious mononucleosis negative; serologic tests rule out cytomegalovirus infection and toxoplasmosis.
Imaging	Angio: presence of **coronary artery aneurysms.**
Gross Pathology	Aneurysmal dilatation of the coronary arteries.
Micro Pathology	Coronary arteritis is usually demonstrated at autopsy together with aneurysm formation and thrombosis.
Treatment	Aspirin and IV gamma globulin are effective in preventing coronary complications if initiated early.
Discussion	The disease is usually self-limited, but in a few instances fatal coronary thrombosis has occurred during the acute stage of the disease or many months after apparently complete recovery. Case-fatality rates have been about 1%–2%.

· ·

KAWASAKI'S SYNDROME

ID/CC	A 30-year-old **woman** is seen with an **itchy rash** over her **wrists**, her **forearms**, and the **inner aspects of her thighs**.
HPI	She complains that fresh **lesions occur along scratch marks and areas of trauma** (= KOEBNER'S PHENOMENON).
PE	VS: no fever. PE: polygonal, **purple, flat-topped papules and plaques; tiny white dots and lines over papules** (= WICKHAM'S STRIAE); white netlike pattern of **lesions over oral mucosa**.
Labs	N/A
Imaging	N/A
Gross Pathology	Flat-topped, violaceous papules and plaques **without scales**.
Micro Pathology	Dense, **bandlike (lichenoid) lymphocytic infiltrate** (predominantly T cells) within upper dermis, obscuring the dermal–epidermal interface; **sawtooth pattern of rete ridges**; degeneration of basal cells with fibrillary bodies.
Treatment	**Steroids**, topical (potent fluorinated) or systemic; **isotretinoin** is an effective alternative, but risk of **teratogenicity** must be borne in mind when prescribing.
Discussion	A **self-limited inflammatory skin** disease, often with hyperpigmented areas when the inflammation subsides after one or two years.

· ·

LICHEN PLANUS

ID/CC	A 25-year-old male is admitted to the hospital for an evaluation of **recurrent epistaxis.**
HPI	The patient's mother died of a **massive pulmonary hemorrhage due to an arteriovenous malformation.**
PE	**Small telangiectatic lesions** seen on lips, oral and nasal mucosa, tongue, and tips of fingers and toes; anemia noted; no pulmonary bruit heard (to detect an AV malformation).
Labs	CBC: normocytic, normochromic anemia (due to occult gastrointestinal blood loss).
Imaging	CT: AV malformations in liver and spleen.
Gross Pathology	N/A
Micro Pathology	N/A
Treatment	**Estrogens** may be tried to control recurrent epistaxis; significant visceral AV malformations may require embolization.
Discussion	Hereditary hemorrhagic telangiectasia is inherited as an **autosomal-dominant trait.** Telangiectasias may first be seen during adolescence and then increase in incidence with age, peaking between the ages of 45 and 60 years.

· ·

OSLER–WEBER–RENDU SYNDROME

ID/CC	A **45-year-old woman** visits her dermatologist complaining of **painful, blistering skin lesions over her back, chest, and arms that break down and leave denuded skin areas.**
HPI	Over the past few years she has had **large recurrent aphthous ulcers in the mouth.** She was not taking any drugs before her symptoms developed.
PE	**Large aphthous ulcers** seen over oral and vaginal mucosa; **vesiculobullous skin lesions** seen in **various stages;** vertical pressure over bullae leads to **lateral extension** (= "BULLA SPREAD SIGN"); skin over bullae **peels like that of a "hot tomato"** (= NIKOLSKY'S SIGN).
Labs	Indirect immunofluorescence test to detect antibodies in serum shows presence of IgG antibodies.
Imaging	N/A
Gross Pathology	Fresh vesicle is selected for biopsy.
Micro Pathology	Lesions show loss of **cohesion of epidermal cells** (= ACANTHOLYSIS) that produces clefts directly above basal cell layer; Tzanck smear of material from floor of a bulla reveals acantholytic cells that are round with large hyperchromatic nuclei and homogeneous cytoplasm; **direct immunofluorescence** reveals **characteristic intercellular staining.**
Treatment	Steroids are mainstay of therapy; cytotoxic drugs (cyclophosphamide).
Discussion	Pemphigus vulgaris, an intraepidermal blistering disease of the skin and mucous membranes, usually appears in individuals in the third to fifth decade of life. The blisters result from loss of adhesion between epidermal cells caused by the production of autoantibodies that are directed against keratinocyte cell surface proteins; loss of cell–cell contact between desmosomes (which are sites of attachment for epidermal cells) has been demonstrated by electron microscopy.

. . . .

PEMPHIGUS

ID/CC	A 40-year-old male comes to a dermatology outpatient clinic with an extensive, mildly pruritic and chronic skin rash.
HPI	**It improves during the summer and markedly worsens in cold weather.** The patient was previously diagnosed by an orthopedic surgeon with **distal interphalangeal joint arthropathy.**
PE	Multiple salmon-colored plaques with overlying silvery scales seen over back and extensor aspects of upper and lower limbs; on removing scale, **underlying pinpoint bleeding capillaries** seen (= AUSPITZ SIGN); lesions seen at places aligned along scratch marks (= KOEBNER PHENOMENA); **pitting of nails** with occasional onycholysis seen.
Labs	N/A
Imaging	XR-Hands: asymmetric degenerative changes involving the distal interphalangeal joints, with **"pencil-in-cup"** deformity.
Gross Pathology	N/A
Micro Pathology	Skin biopsy reveals markedly thickened stratum corneum with layered zones of parakeratosis (retention of nuclei); markedly hyperplastic epidermis with broadening of rete projections; intracorneal or subcorneal collections of PMNs (= MUNRO'S MICROABSCESSES); **marked degree of epidermal hyperplasia with little inflammatory infiltrate** (characteristic microscopic finding).
Treatment	Exposure to sunlight; the following have been used either alone or in combination: tar ointment, dithranol, PUVA, topical steroids, and cytotoxic drugs such as methotrexate.
Discussion	Psoriasis is a genetically determined condition that is characterized by well-defined plaques covered by silvery scales. Lesions are most commonly seen in an extensor distribution, but the nails, scalp, palms, and soles may also be involved; arthritis of the distal interphalangeal joint may be seen in 20% of cases.

· ·

PSORIASIS

ID/CC	A 19-year-old **black male** complains of **unsightly white** (depigmented) **patches** on his knees and elbows (bony prominences).
HPI	He has no history of associated **pruritus** or **discomfort**. The first patch appeared over the left elbow a few months ago, and the process has been **progressive** since then.
PE	PE: flat, well-demarcated areas of **depigmentation** on face (perioral or periocular), elbows, knees, and neck and in skin folds; sites of recent skin trauma are also seen to have **undergone depigmentation** (= KOEBNER'S PHENOMENON); **most hairs within vitiliginous patch are white.**
Labs	N/A
Imaging	N/A
Gross Pathology	N/A
Micro Pathology	**Absent melanin pigment** on skin biopsy stain with ferric ferricyanide; **absence of melanocytes** on electron microscopy.
Treatment	No established satisfactory treatment exists; a promising approach is oral psoralen (photosensitizing drug) followed by exposure to artificial long-wave ultraviolet light (UVA); potent fluorinated steroid topically may be helpful. Generalized vitiligo may be treated by depigmentation of normal skin.
Discussion	Vitiligo usually appears in otherwise-healthy persons, but several systemic disorders occur more often in patients with vitiligo, including thyroid disease (e.g., hyperthyroidism, Graves' disease and thyroiditis), Addison's disease, pernicious anemia, alopecia areata, uveitis, and diabetes mellitus. Vitiligo may be inherited as an **autosomal-dominant trait** with incomplete penetrance and variable expression. Most studies, however, point to an **autoimmune** basis (circulating complement binding anti-melanocyte antibodies have been detected).

· ·

VITILIGO

ID/CC	A 58-year-old male complains of **headache,** anxiety, and increased sleepiness (= SOMNOLENCE) while experiencing an **acute exacerbation of COPD.**
HPI	The patient is a **chronic smoker** and also complains of recent **blurring of vision.** He has a history of episodic shortness of breath, mucoid cough, and occasional wheezing (consistent with predominantly **bronchitic COPD**) but no history of neurologic deficit, previous hypertension, or diabetes.
PE	VS: tachycardia; tachypnea; mild systolic hypertension; no fever. PE: anxious and in moderate respiratory distress; using accessory muscles of respiration with prolonged expiration; mild **central cyanosis and pallor; no clubbing;** extremities warm; **flapping tremor of hand** (= ASTERIXIS); **bounding pulses** (due to high volume); funduscopy reveals **early papilledema;** chest barrel-shaped with bilateral rhonchi and occasional rales; no focal neurologic deficits.
Labs	ABGs: **hypoxia, hypercapnia, and partially compensated respiratory acidosis.** CBC: polycythemia.
Imaging	CXR (PA view): increased bronchovascular markings (dirty lung fields).
Gross Pathology	N/A
Micro Pathology	N/A
Treatment	**Low-dose continuous oxygen inhalation and, if required, mechanical ventilation** to reverse acidosis; antibiotics, bronchodilators, and steroids are used in COPD patients.
Discussion	Hypercapnia produces a variety of neurologic abnormalities; initial symptoms include headache, somnolence, blurred vision, restlessness, and anxiety that can progress to tremors, asterixis, delirium, and coma.

· ·

CARBON DIOXIDE NARCOSIS

ID/CC   A 20-year-old college student is brought back from a summer camp in the mountains after developing **severe shortness of breath** (= DYSPNEA), cough with **blood-tinged sputum** (= HEMOPTYSIS), and wheezing.

HPI   The group had **ascended to a height** of 8,000 feet and had engaged in **strenuous physical activities**. The patient subsequently developed dyspnea and cough that worsened during the night, leading to **marked respiratory distress and a shock-like state.**

PE   VS: tachycardia; tachypnea; hypotension. PE: **central cyanosis;** pale and cold extremities; marked **respiratory distress; widespread rales and rhonchi** over both lung fields.

Labs   CBC: **elevated hematocrit and hemoglobin;** mildly increased WBC. ABGs: markedly **decreased arterial PO_2; low PCO_2. Increased pH.** ECG: sinus tachycardia with **acute pulmonary hypertension.**

Imaging   CXR (PA view): **noncardiogenic pulmonary edema** and prominent main pulmonary artery.

Gross Pathology   N/A

Micro Pathology   Extensive pulmonary edema; protein-rich exudate with alveolar hemorrhages and **alveolar hyaline membranes;** dilatation of right ventricle.

Treatment   **Prompt descent, hyperbaric oxygen inhalation, sublingual nifedipine (after checking blood pressure),** placement in **portable hyperbaric chamber** while being transported; hospital management comprises **continuous high-flow oxygen, steroids for CNS symptoms, and acetazolamide.**

Discussion   High-altitude pulmonary edema is primarily a disorder of the pulmonary circulation **induced by sustained alveolar hypoxia.** The initiating event is an abnormal degree of **hypoxia induced pulmonary arteriolar (precapillary) constriction** (hypoxia causes dilatation of systemic blood vessels) that elevates pulmonary arterial pressure. The combination of **increased blood flow** and pressure causes the arterioles to dilate, resulting in **edema.**

. . . .

HIGH-ALTITUDE SICKNESS

ID/CC   A 28-year-old woman **found on a park bench apparently dead** is brought to the ER in the early hours of the morning.

HPI   No discernible pulse was palpated, but a **faint, infrequent respiratory effort was noted**; CPR was begun and continued during her transport to the hospital. The **temperature overnight was near-freezing** with continuous rain.

PE   VS: arterial **pulse not palpated**; hypotension; reduced respiratory rate; **severe hypothermia (< 28 C)**. PE: no respiratory effort; **fixed and dilated pupils**; blotchy areas of erythema on skin; bullae over buttocks; chest exam shows diffuse rales bilaterally; absent bowel sounds; absent deep tendon reflexes.

Labs   CBC: raised hematocrit; hypoglycemia; BUN and creatinine raised, bicarbonate depressed, hyperkalemia. ABGs: severe metabolic acidosis. ECG: evidence of **marked bradycardia with Osborn (or J) waves.**

Imaging   CXR: patchy atelectasis.

Gross Pathology   N/A

Micro Pathology   N/A

Treatment   Intubation and ventilation as necessary; cardiac massage for arrest; warm the patient through use of a combination of heated blankets, heat packs, warm gastric lavage, warm-water immersion, high-flow oxygen and IV hypotonic dextrose.

Discussion   Hypothermia is defined as core temperature below 35 C; **severe accidental hypothermia (below 30 C, or 86 F) is associated with marked depression in cerebral blood flow and cerebral oxygen requirement, reduced cardiac output, and decreased arterial pressure.** Victims can **appear to be lifeless** as a result of marked depression of brain function. Peripheral pulses may be difficult to detect because of bradycardia and vasoconstriction.

. . . .

HYPOTHERMIA

ID/CC	A 25-year-old male is brought to the ER after sustaining a stab wound on his left thigh following a drunken brawl.
HPI	A tourniquet was tied above the site, which the attendants said was **spurting blood like "a tap run open."**
PE	VS: hypotension; weak, fast pulse. PE: anxious; **cool skin with reduced capillary filling;** very low central venous pressure; releasing tourniquet confirmed femoral artery puncture.
Labs	CBC: mildly decreased hematocrit; BUN and creatinine normal; lytes normal.
Imaging	Arteriogram shows abrupt termination of dye propagation in the common femoral artery.
Gross Pathology	N/A
Micro Pathology	N/A
Treatment	Arrest of femoral artery hemorrhage with vascular repair; intensive IV fluid therapy using human albumin solutions, normal saline, and cross-matched blood transfusions; close monitoring of pulse rate, blood pressure, urine output, and central venous pressure.
Discussion	The clinical conditions that cause hypovolemic shock include **acute and subacute hemorrhage and dehydration;** fluid loss into an extravascular compartment can significantly reduce intravascular volume and result in nonhemorrhagic hypovolemic shock. Acute pancreatitis, loss of the enteral integument (from conditions such as burns and surgical wounds), or occlusive or dynamic ileus can all induce oligemic hypotension as a result of extravasation of fluids into the extracellular compartment. Other forms of water and solute loss, such as diarrhea, hyperglycemia (leading to glucosuria), diabetes insipidus, salt-wasting nephritis, protracted vomiting, adrenocortical failure, acute peritonitis, and overzealous use of diuretics, can also lead to decreased intravascular volume and hypovolemic shock.

. . . .

HYPOVOLEMIC SHOCK

ID/CC	A 30-year-old male complains of progressive weakness and fatigue over the past two years.
HPI	Over the past year, he has had loss of appetite and weight loss; he also has frequent vomiting and an almost constant feeling of nausea. His wife noted that he is excessively irritable and restless.
PE	VS: hypotension. PE: **diffuse dark-brown hyperpigmentation,** especially about the elbows, around the areolae, and along palmar creases; hyperpigmented bluish-black patches on oral mucosa.
Labs	CBC: **eosinophilia. ACTH stimulation test diagnostic, demonstrating failure of cortisol level to rise.** Lytes: hyperkalemia; hyponatremia. ABGs: mild metabolic acidosis. **Hypoglycemia;** high ACTH levels following cosyntropin administration localizes disease to adrenals.
Imaging	CT Scan- Abd: small adrenal glands (autoimmune) or enlarged adrenal glands (inflammatory, hemorrhagic and metastatic causes).
Gross Pathology	Bilateral atrophic adrenal glands.
Micro Pathology	Fibrosis, atrophy and diffuse lymphocytic infiltration of the adrenal glands.
Treatment	Replacement therapy with glucocorticoids and mineralocorticoids.
Discussion	Addison's disease has two main origins: granulomatous infections such as tuberculosis and histoplasmosis (responsible for a minority of cases in the U.S.) and the more common cause—an autoimmune disorder in which lymphocytic and plasma cell invasion of the adrenal is accompanied by antiadrenal antibodies in the plasma. Adrenal insufficiency can complicate AIDS, as the adrenals may be infiltrated by opportunistic pathogens (such as CMV) and by Kaposi's sarcoma. Metastasis to the adrenals and disseminated meningococcal infection (Waterhouse–Friderichsen syndrome) are other causes; drugs such as ketoconazole and etomidate may also cause adrenal insufficiency. **FIRST AID** p.239

. . . .

ADDISON'S DISEASE

ID/CC	A 40-year-old **woman** is seen in the outpatient clinic with complaint of sudden-onset **painful neck swelling.**
HPI	Prior to this she had a **sore throat, malaise, and fever.** Pain over the thyroid area radiates to the ears and is worse on swallowing.
PE	VS: fever; tachycardia. PE: fine **tremors** of tongue and fingers of outstretched hands; firm, exquisitely **tender, diffuse, mildly enlarged goiter** palpable; nonfirm nodularity felt; no cervical lymphadenopathy; no ophthalmopathy (distinguishes from Graves').
Labs	CBC: elevated leukocytes. Elevated ESR (characteristic); elevated free T3 and T4 levels and resin uptake (seen only during early stages due to follicular disruption and hormone release; later transient hypothyroidism may ensue; rarely permanent hypothyroidism results); depressed TSH; markedly **reduced radioactive iodine uptake** (key diagnostic feature and used for differentiating it from Graves' disease).
Imaging	Nuc: poorly visualized thyroid gland.
Gross Pathology	Diffusely enlarged thyroid gland; involved areas are firm and yellow against the normal uninvolved brown thyroid substance.
Micro Pathology	Early lesions include **disruption of thyroid follicles with a neutrophilic infiltrate and formation of microabscesses;** subsequently **multinucleated giant cells** may be seen surrounding colloid fragments, resembling granulomas.
Treatment	**Propranolol and analgesics** for symptomatic relief are generally adequate; condition is **self-limiting** in 6–8 weeks; severe cases may require **prednisone** therapy; permanent hypothyroidism may result on rare occasions, in which case hormone replacement is required. **Antithyroid drugs are not indicated.**
Discussion	De Quervain's or subacute **painful** thyroiditis is the most common cause of severe thyroid pain and tenderness; it is most common in **women 20–50 years** of age and shows an association with **HLA-B35.** Its exact etiology is unknown.

DE QUERVAIN'S THYROIDITIS

ID/CC	A **30-year-old woman** presents with complaints of excessive **anxiety, tremors, bulging of the eyeballs** (= EXOPHTHALMOS), and a progressively increasing neck mass (= GOITER).
HPI	She has had significant **weight loss** over the past few months **despite an increased appetite.** She also reports **excessive bleeding during menses** (= MENORRHAGIA).
PE	VS: **tachycardia.** PE: anxious; Eye exam reveals **bilateral exophthalmos, lid lag, "stare"** (due to lid retraction), **and convergence weakness;** smooth, nontender diffuse **goitre; bruit** over thyroid; no cervical lymphadenopathy; fine **tremor** of fingers of outstretched hands; **onycholysis and palmar erythema** (= THYROID ACROPACHY); nontender **purplish edematous plaques on shin** (= PRETIBIAL MYXEDEMA).
Labs	CBC: normocytic, normochromic anemia. **Elevated T4 and T3 levels; TSH levels undetectable; elevated thyroid-stimulating immunoglobulin (TSI)** (TSH receptor antibody that stimulates thyroid hormone production).
Imaging	Nuc: diffusely increased radioactive iodine uptake.
Gross Pathology	Gland moderately and diffusely enlarged and meaty red-brown; normal waxy appearance lost (due to loss of colloid).
Micro Pathology	**Hyperplasia of follicular epithelial cells;** colloid absent or greatly reduced.
Treatment	**Radioactive iodine or thionamides** (methimazole and propylthiouracil) are treatment of choice; radioactive iodine cannot be used in pregnancy; **subtotal thyroidectomy** required in selected cases; beta-blockers such as **propranolol** provide symptomatic relief.
Discussion	Graves' is an **autoimmune disease** that presents as a toxic diffuse **goiter associated with ophthalmopathy** (exophthalmos) and **dermopathy** (pretibial myxedema).

· ·

HYPERTHYROIDISM (GRAVES' DISEASE)

ID/CC	A 7-year-old male is brought to a physician for an evaluation of precocious puberty.
HPI	He has a history of severe headaches and visual blurring.
PE	Fully developed secondary sexual characteristics (Tanner stage IV); paralysis of upward gaze (= PARINAUD SYNDROME); convergence retraction nystagmus; funduscopy reveals bilateral papilledema.
Labs	Normal lab parameters.
Imaging	MR-Head: obstructive hydrocephalus and brightly enhancing mass in region of pineal gland.
Gross Pathology	N/A
Micro Pathology	Microscopic pathology reveals tumor to be of germ cell origin (= GERMINOMA).
Treatment	Neurosurgery and radiation therapy are mainstay of treatment.
Discussion	Pineal region tumors include pineocytomas and pineoblastomas derived from the pineal parenchymal cells as well as teratomas and germinomas; precocious puberty occurs in young males, primarily as a result of destruction of the pineal gland by a germinoma.

· ·

PINEALOMA

ID/CC	A 40-year-old woman complains of an unsightly, **progressively increasing neck swelling** and intermittent shortness of breath.
HPI	She has noticed unusually **engorged neck veins** and has recently developed **difficulty swallowing solids** (= DYSPHAGIA) and **loud snoring** (= STRIDOR) while sleeping. There are **no symptoms of hypothyroidism or hyperthyroidism.** She uses iodized salt (iodine deficiency produces endemic goiter).
PE	PE: anterior, **irregular-surfaced swelling that moves with deglutition** (= MULTINODULAR GOITER); percussion over sternum is dull (due to retrosternal extension of goiter); **suffusion of face with marked dyspnea when patient raises both arms** overhead for a few seconds (due to tracheal compression); **no tremors or eye signs;** no cervical adenopathy.
Labs	T3, T4 normal; TSH elevated; thyroid autoantibodies absent.
Imaging	CXR: **retrosternal extension** of the goiter, producing tracheal compression and deviation. US/CT: **diffuse multinodularity.**
Gross Pathology	Resected **thyroid grossly enlarged;** surface **covered by nodules of varying sizes.**
Micro Pathology	Follicles **distended with colloid;** follicle lining cells flattened; degenerative changes present in between nodules.
Treatment	**Subtotal thyroidectomy; thyroxine** subsequently administered to **suppress** TSH levels and prevent recurrence.
Discussion	The cause of enlargement of the thyroid is most often unknown; known causes include **iodine deficiency** (in endemic areas), **ingestion of goitrogens** (e.g., cabbage, cassava), or **defects** in the synthesis or transport of hormone.

. . . .

SPORADIC MULTINODULAR GOITER

ID/CC	A 40-year-old **male** presents with complaints of increasing **yellowness** of his eyes and skin, **darkly colored urine,** and loss of appetite.
HPI	He has no history of blood transfusions, contact with other jaundiced persons, or exposure to an epidemic of hepatitis in the neighborhood; the patient is a known **alcoholic.**
PE	Icterus; parotid enlargement, **Dupuytren's contracture** in left index and little finger; **palmar erythema;** mildly **tender hepatomegaly;** no splenomegaly or ascites.
Labs	CBC: anemia; leukocytosis. Elevated serum bilirubin; **elevated AST and ALT (AST > ALT)** (typically seen in alcoholic liver disease; in other parenchymal liver diseases, ALT is more elevated); increased alkaline phosphatase and gamma-glutamyl-transferase (GGT); serologic markers for hepatitis A, B and C negative.
Imaging	US-Abdomen: hepatomegaly with coarsened echo texture suggestive of hepatitis and fatty infiltration.
Gross Pathology	Enlarged liver with yellow and greasy surface (shrunken size with micronodular surface is seen in cirrhotic stage).
Micro Pathology	**Hepatocellular necrosis, neutrophilic infiltration, and alcoholic hyaline bodies** (= MALLORY BODIES); some hepatocytes distended with fat, displacing nucleus to side. Perivenular and sinusoidal fibrosis also seen.
Treatment	Abstinence is most effective; nutritional support; colchicine tried with variable success.
Discussion	Liver disease produced by excessive consumption of ethanol includes fatty liver, alcoholic hepatitis, and cirrhosis; fatty change and, to an extent, alcoholic hepatitis may reverse fully with abstinence. 10-15% of chronic alcoholics develop cirrhosis.

ALCOHOLIC HEPATITIS

ID/CC	A 50-year-old male presents with a long-standing history of **retrosternal burning, belching, and water brash.**
HPI	He is a **chronic smoker and alcoholic** and is under treatment for **gastroesophageal reflux dyspepsia.**
PE	Physical exam normal.
Labs	UGI endoscopy reveals linear streaks of red, velvety mucosa at gastroesophageal junction.
Imaging	Barium swallow: fine reticular pattern distal to an esophageal stricture; gastroesophageal reflux.
Gross Pathology	**Red, velvety mucosa in form of circumferential band and linear streaks around gastroesophageal junction.**
Micro Pathology	Mixture of **metaplastic gastric and intestinal-type columnar epithelial cells** (mucin-secreting and absorptive, respectively).
Treatment	Antireflux medication (Cisapride); proton pump inhibitors and antacids; cessation of smoking and alcohol; careful follow-up to detect esophageal cancer.
Discussion	Barrett's esophagus is marked by **metaplasia of the distal esophageal squamous epithelium to a columnar epithelium in response to prolonged injury;** long-standing esophageal reflux leads to inflammation and ulceration of squamous mucosa. Healing occurs through reepithelialization by pluripotent cells, which in the setting of low pH differentiate into the more resistant gastric (both cardiac and fundic) type or the specialized columnar (intestinal) type. Only the columnar type is of clinical importance. The most serious complication is the development of **adenocarcinoma;** hence, patients with Barrett's should undergo endoscopic surveillance.

. . . .

BARRETT'S ESOPHAGUS

ID/CC	A 40-year-old woman is seen with complaints of sudden-onset, progressively increasing **abdominal distention and pain** and **vomiting**.
HPI	The patient also complains of **visible abdominal and back veins** that appear while she is **standing** and **look like ropes**. In addition, she has observed **increasing swelling of her feet**. She has been taking **oral contraceptives** for a few years.
PE	Icterus; **pitting pedal edema**; markedly distended abdomen;. dilated, tortuous veins over abdomen and back; **flow is from below upward** (due to hepatic vein and IVC obstruction); **hepatojugular reflux absent**; fluid thrill but shifting dullness present (ascites); mildly tender **hepatomegaly** and **splenomegaly**.
Labs	CBC: leukocytosis. LFTs elevated; ascitic fluid **transudative**.
Imaging	US-Abdomen: hepatosplenomegaly and ascites. US-Doppler: increased portal vein flow; **hepatic veins obstructed where they empty into the inferior vena cava**. IVC portovenography: confirms obstruction.
Gross Pathology	Thrombosis of hepatic vein where it drains into the inferior vena cava. Liver is swollen and reddish-purple and has a tense capsule.
Micro Pathology	Affected areas show severe centrilobular congestion and necrosis.
Treatment	Balloon angioplasty; thrombolytic therapy into hepatic veins; surgical removal or bypass of the obstruction; **stop oral contraceptives**.
Discussion	This syndrome occurs with conditions that predispose to thrombosis, e.g., polycythemia vera, pregnancy, postpartum states, use of oral contraceptives, PNH, and intra-abdominal cancers; membranous webs in the inferior vena cava may produce the obstruction.

· ·

BUDD–CHIARI SYNDROME

ID/CC	A **66-year-old Scandinavian** male comes to the doctor's office for an insurance physical complaining of increasing **fatigue, occasional indigestion, and diarrhea.**
HPI	He has been taking antacids for his dyspepsia.
PE	**Marked pallor; mild splenomegaly.**
Labs	CBC/PBS: **macrocytic anemia.** Low vitamin B_{12} levels; elevated homocystine and methylmalonic acid; **Schilling test confirms vitamin B_{12} malabsorption** corrected with administration of intrinsic factor; **anti-parietal cell antibodies present; reduced gastric acid formation** (= ACHLORHYDRIA); biopsy taken during endoscopy reveals **chronic atrophic gastritis** with no evidence of intestinal metaplasia. Endoscopy: thinning of mucosa and flattening of rugal fold seen more in fundus and body of stomach with **sparing of antrum.**
Imaging	N/A
Gross Pathology	See labs.
Micro Pathology	Lymphocytes and plasma cell infiltrates in lamina propria; decreased number of glands.
Treatment	Parenteral administration of vitamin B_{12}; regular follow-up (chronic atrophic gastritis **predisposes to gastric carcinoma**).
Discussion	Pernicious anemia is characterized by chronic atrophic gastritis with achlorhydria and antibodies to parietal cells and intrinsic factor. **FIRST AID** p.228

. . . .

CHRONIC ATROPHIC GASTRITIS

ID/CC	A 21-year-old female complains of **intermittent abdominal pain, mild, nonbloody diarrhea,** and anorexia of two years' duration.
HPI	During these episodes, she describes that she also has a fever and that the pain is almost always confined to the **right lower abdomen** and is cramping in nature.
PE	Pallor; weight loss; **abdominal mass in right iliac fossa** (thickened bowel loop); **perianal fistulas.**
Labs	CBC: megaloblastic anemia; leukocytosis. **Positive stool guaiac test;** stool exam reveals no parasites.
Imaging	BE: granulomatous colitis and regional enteritis involving multiple areas, most commonly ileum and ascending colon, with intervening segments of normal mucosa.
Gross Pathology	**Terminal ileum** (lesions most commonly seen in ileocecal are, but can affect any part of the GI tract) shows lesions which have a "**cobblestone**" appearance; **discontinuous areas of inflammation, edema, and fibrosis** (= "SKIP LESIONS").
Micro Pathology	**Chronic inflammatory involvement of submucosal layers of bowel wall** (= TRANSMURAL INFLAMMATION), manifested mainly by lymphocytic infiltration with associated lymphoid hyperplasia and formation of noncaseating granulomas.
Treatment	**Antidiarrheal drugs and systemic glucocorticoids; surgery** if patient develops severe malabsorption and subacute intestinal obstruction.
Discussion	Complications include adhesions, ulcers, strictures, fissures, and fistulas. Differentiate from ulcerative colitis. **FIRST AID** p.229

. . . .

CROHN'S DISEASE

ID/CC   A 50-year-old **white male** presents to a dermatology clinic with complaints of **painless** fragile skin and boils on the **back** of his hands and forearms with dark scars (= HYPERPIGMENTATION) after rupture and healing.

HPI   Lately he has noticed **dark brown (may also be red-orange) urine after prolonged standing.** His **father had a similar skin ailment** (20% of cases are autosomal dominant). He claims to be taking no drugs and notes that the boils **became worse after a drinking binge.**

PE   VS: normal. PE: **vesicles and bullae** on **dorsal surface** of hands and forearms (classic **photosensitive distribution**); hypertrichosis and hyperpigmentation over involved areas; striking degree of thickening, scarring, and calcification (= PSEUDOSCLERODERMA) of affected areas; moderate nontender hepatomegaly.

Labs   Dramatically increased **uroporphyrin and 7-carboxylate porphyrin in urine and increased isocoproporphyrin in feces** (diagnostic); urinary ALT and porphobilinogen normal; plasma porphyrin levels elevated; LFTs elevated; viral serology reveals **hepatitis C infection** (highly associated); **increased total iron-binding capacity saturation** and serum iron (due to iron overload); **deficiency of liver uroporphyrinogen decarboxylase.**

Imaging   US/CT-Abdomen: hepatomegaly.

Gross Pathology   Moderately enlarged liver.

Micro Pathology   **Siderosis, liver cell necrosis, and inflammation** on liver biopsy; **fluorescent porphyrin pigment** on liver histology; fluorescent porphyrin pigment on liver and skin biopsy.

Treatment   **Phlebotomy; discontinue alcohol; avoid iron supplements;** consider **low-dose oral chloroquine** (high or usual dose may exacerbate photosensitivity). Avoid sun exposure.

Discussion   Porphyria cutanea tarda (PCT) is the **most common porphyria,** predominantly occurring in male Caucasians and rarely affecting blacks. It may develop after **exposure to estrogens or exogenous chemicals** (e.g., **hexachlorobenzene,** a fungicide).

· ·

PORPHYRIA CUTANEA TARDA

ID/CC	A 55-year-old **woman** presents with increasing yellowing of the eyes (= JAUNDICE), fatigue, and **chronic itching.**
HPI	She also has **rheumatoid arthritis and chronic thyroiditis.** She has no prior history of jaundice, does not drink alcohol, and has never received a blood transfusion.
PE	**Icterus;** numerous scratch marks and excoriations on the skin; xanthomas and **xanthelasma;** hepatomegaly, splenomegaly, and no ascites; rheumatoid joint deformities and goiter (due to chronic thyroiditis).
Labs	Raised ESR; **markedly elevated alkaline phosphatase;** mildly elevated direct bilirubin and aminotransferases; **elevated serum cholesterol** (> 300 mg/dL); serum **antimitochondrial antibody** present in high titer.
Imaging	US-Abdomen: hepatomegaly and splenomegaly.
Gross Pathology	Dark green, enlarged liver (in late stages, liver shows cirrhosis which cannot be distinguished from other causes).
Micro Pathology	Bile duct destruction with lymphocytic–plasmacytic infiltration of portal areas; **periportal epithelioid granuloma formation** and portal scarring with linking of portal tracts; periportal bile stasis noted (in advanced cases, cirrhosis may be found).
Treatment	Cholestyramine to control pruritus; immunosuppression; liver transplantation is the only definitive treatment.
Discussion	Primary biliary cirrhosis is a chronic liver disease of probable **autoimmune** etiology that occurs primarily in **middle-aged women** and is characterized by **nonsuppurative obliterative cholangitis that progresses to cirrhosis;** it is associated with other autoimmune diseases in 85% of cases. Complications include cirrhosis and portal hypertension, malabsorption due to steatorrhea, and osteoporosis due to malabsorption of vitamin D and calcium.

· ·

PRIMARY BILIARY CIRRHOSIS

ID/CC	A 31-year-old male complains of having more than five bowel movements a day together with **cramping abdominal pain** and **tenesmus**.
HPI	The patient adds that his stools consist of watery or pasty material with **mucus** and gross quantities of **blood**. He also complains of intermittent fatigue, fever, and an increased need for sleep.
PE	VS: mild fever. PE: localized tenderness over distal colon.
Labs	CBC: anemia; leukocytosis. Elevated ESR; stool exam reveals **no parasites; no bacterial pathogen** isolated in culture.
Imaging	BE: early mucosal granularity; later, rigidity and **loss of haustrations** (= "LEAD PIPE"), with ragged ulcerated mucosa and ulcerations. Colonoscopy: **mucosal erythema and granularity** with hemorrhaging and **inflammatory polyps.**
Gross Pathology	Scarring and coarse, granular mucosal surface indicating presence of microulcerations; mucosal surface is friable; **lesions are continuous** from anal to oral direction.
Micro Pathology	Increased numbers of lymphocytes, plasma cells, and PMNs; atrophy of mucosal glands and presence of PMNs in crypts of Lieberkühn (often called crypt abscesses).
Treatment	Antidiarrheal drugs; sulfasalazine, 5-ASA preparations; glucocorticoids; surgery if indicated.
Discussion	Patients with this disease are at **increased risk for colon cancer.** Factors favoring the development of colon cancer in ulcerative colitis are the duration of disease for eight years or longer, involvement of the entire colon, continuous clinical activity, and, possibly, a severe initial attack. It is routinely advised that patients undergo regular surveillance that includes colonoscopy and an examination of multiple biopsies for dysplastic changes or frank cancer. Another major complication is massive intestinal hemorrhage with shock and sepsis. **FIRST AID** p.229

. . . .

ULCERATIVE COLITIS

ID/CC	A 35-year-old woman is admitted to the hospital with **left-sided weakness upon awakening.**
HPI	She has **no history** of prior headaches, seizures, hypertension, or diabetes and neither smokes nor takes drugs. Her **first three pregnancies** were **spontaneously aborted;** the fourth resulted in **unexpected fetal death.**
PE	VS: normal. PE: patient conscious; mild pallor; **left hemiplegia** with exaggerated deep tendon reflexes and extensor plantar response (= POSITIVE BABINSKI'S SIGN); no neck rigidity; fundus normal; no carotid bruit; no cardiac murmurs; **reddish-blue mottling of skin in fishnet pattern** (= LIVEDO RETICULARIS) on extremities; positive Homans' sign in left leg.
Labs	CBC: mild thrombocytopenia. **Prolonged PTT and PT;** normal bleeding and clotting times; **false-positive VDRL** (titer < 1:18); FTA-ABS for syphilis negative; ELISA shows presence of **anticardiolipin antibody (ACA).**
Imaging	CT-Head (24 hours later): hypodensity (due to infarct) in right internal capsule.
Gross Pathology	N/A
Micro Pathology	N/A
Treatment	**Anticoagulant therapy** with heparin; use of **low-dose aspirin and heparin,** either alone or in combination with **prednisone,** is advocated during pregnancy in cases with a **complicated obstetric history** (e.g., spontaneous abortions or intrauterine demise).
Discussion	The presence of **lupus anticoagulant** and **ACA** defines antiphospholipid syndrome; it is further characterized by **recurrent deep venous thrombosis** in the lower extremities, thrombosis in the renal and hepatic veins, **pulmonary hypertension, cerebral artery occlusion** associated with stroke and transient ischemic attacks (TIAs), and neurologic findings that resemble multi-infarct dementia or epilepsy.

· ·

ANTIPHOSPHOLIPID ANTIBODY SYNDROME

ID/CC	An 11-month-old male presents with marked **pallor, failure to thrive, and delayed developmental motor milestones.**
HPI	The child's parents are **Indian** immigrants.
PE	Marked pallor; mild icterus; frontal bossing and **maxillary hypertrophy** (= "CHIPMUNK FACIES"); **splenomegaly.**
Labs	CBC: severe microcytic, hypochromic anemia with **anisopoikilocytosis;** decreased reticulocyte count (ineffective erythropoiesis). **HbA absent; HbF 95%;** mildly increased unconjugated bilirubin.
Imaging	XR-Skull (lateral): maxillary overgrowth and widening of diploic spaces with **"hair on end" appearance** of frontal bone, caused by vertical trabeculae.
Gross Pathology	Expansion of hematopoietic bone marrow causing thinning of cortical bone or new bone formation.
Micro Pathology	Red marrow increased; yellow marrow decreased; marked erythroid hyperplasia in marrow (ineffective erythropoiesis).
Treatment	**Blood transfusion, folic acid supplement, iron chelation therapy** with desferrioxamine to reverse hemosiderosis, **bone marrow transplantation** using HLA-matched sibling donors.
Discussion	Beta-thalassemia results from decreased synthesis of beta-globin chains due to errors in transcription and translation of mRNA. Alpha-thalassemia results from decreased synthesis of alpha-globin chains due to deletion of one or more of the four alpha genes that are normally present. **FIRST AID** p.226

· ·

BETA-THALASSEMIA

ID/CC   A **60-year-old male** is referred to an allergist for late-onset **asthma** that has been **unresponsive to bronchodilators and antibiotics.**

HPI   He has also been having chest pain (= ANGINA) and pain in both calves (= CLAUDICATION) on exertion which are of recent onset.

PE   VS: tachypnea; mild fever; **mild hypertension** (BP 150/100) (secondary to renal vascular involvement). PE: marked respiratory distress; widespread **wheezes** bilaterally; numerous **purpuric lesions on feet** (due to cutaneous small vessel vasculitis).

Labs   CBC: mild anemia; leukocytosis (> 10,000/uL); Hct < 35%; thrombocytosis (> 400,000/uL); **eosinophilia (> 1000/uL).** Elevated BUN and creatinine. UA: **proteinuria;** presence of RBCs, WBCs, and **granular casts.** PFTs: FEV_1/FVC ratio reduced (**obstructive pulmonary disease**). ECG: sinus tachycardia.

Imaging   CXR: **bilateral upper and lower lobe infiltrates** and noncavitating nodules.

Gross Pathology   Lung shows hemorrhagic infarcts secondary to thrombi in affected arteries.

Micro Pathology   Transbronchial lung biopsy shows **granulomatous lesions in vascular and extravascular sites accompanied by intense eosinophilia;** skin biopsy of purpuric lesions shows **vasculitic lesions**—fibrinoid necrosis of media with mixture of inflammatory cells extending along adventitia; occasional aneurysms and secondary thromboses seen; the arterial internal elastic lamina is destroyed and intima and media are thickened.

Treatment   **Prednisolone** effective in inducing remission; **cyclophosphamide** used in those **refractory** to steroids; monitor disease course using **ESR levels.**

Discussion   Churg–Strauss is an idiopathic systemic **small- and medium-vessel granulomatous vasculitis** (grouped with polyarteritis nodosa [PAN], which does not involve lungs) characterized by a triad of late-onset **asthma,** a fluctuating **eosinophilia,** and an **extrapulmonary vasculitis.**

· ·

CHURG–STRAUSS SYNDROME

ID/CC A 35-year-old man complains of **pain in his calf muscles while walking** that is **relieved by rest** (= INTERMITTENT CLAUDICATION) together with exertional chest pain.

HPI He has a family history of **premature atherosclerotic coronary artery disease (CAD).**

PE VS: mild hypertension. PE: **obese; palmar xanthomas** and tendon xanthomas; **orange-yellow discoloration of palmar creases** (pathognomonic for **dysbetalipoproteinemia); tuboeruptive xanthomas** on pressure sites (elbows, buttocks, and knees); weak peripheral pulses.

Labs LFTs normal; lipid profile reveals **elevated total cholesterol, triglycerides, and VLDL and reduced LDL and HDL;** electrophoresis reveals **beta migrating VLDL;** isoelectric focusing shows **EII/EII genotype** (nearly pathognomonic).

Imaging Angio-Coronary: atherosclerotic coronary artery disease confirmed.

Gross Pathology Yellowish intraluminal atherosclerotic plaques seen in the aorta and other large vessels.

Micro Pathology Characteristic atherosclerotic plaques.

Treatment **Weight reduction** to ideal body weight, regular exercise, **avoidance** of alcohol and other triglyceride-raising drugs; low-fat, low-cholesterol **diet;** in resistant cases, **gemfibrozil, high-dose nicotinic acid (niacin), and HMG-CoA reductase** inhibitors (statin drugs) may be used.

Discussion Dysbetalipoproteinemia (= TYPE III HYPERLIPOPROTEINEMIA) is defined as the presence of **VLDL particles that migrate to the beta position on electrophoresis** (normal VLDL particles typically migrate to the pre-beta location). Beta-VLDL particles are chylomicrons and VLDL remnants **caused in part by a mutant apo E** that impairs the hepatic uptake of apoprotein-E-containing lipoproteins.

DYSBETALIPOPROTEINEMIA

ID/CC	A **6-year-old male** is brought to a specialist by his parents due to persistent **pain and tenderness on the right side of his chest** of a few months' duration.
HPI	There is **no history of trauma** to the affected area. The child is otherwise well and is growing normally.
PE	Exquisitely tender site found overlying fourth rib on right side anteriorly; remainder of exam unremarkable.
Labs	Routine lab parameters normal.
Imaging	CXR: **punched-out lesion** in fourth rib on right side.
Gross Pathology	**Intramedullary expanding, eroding lesion.**
Micro Pathology	Brownish granulation tissue containing **abundant foamy histiocytes** and **eosinophils** with leukocytes and giant cells.
Treatment	Lesions resolve spontaneously; surgical curettage may accelerate healing.
Discussion	Eosinophilic granuloma is a type of Langerhans cell histiocytosis; it is an indolent disorder that affects children and young adults, especially males. Solitary bone lesions may be asymptomatic or may cause pain and tenderness and, in some instances, pathologic fracture but without any systemic manifestations. Diagnosis is based on radiographic demonstration of a localized destructive lesion arising from inside the marrow cavity. The **skull, mandible** and **spine** are common locations. In some cases there may be spontaneous healing or fibrosis within a period of 1–2 years.

. . . .

EOSINOPHILIC GRANULOMA

ID/CC   A 12-year-old **black male** complains of **cola-colored urine** and marked fatigue following the administration of **primaquine** for *Plasmodium vivax* malaria.

HPI   When treated with **dapsone** for dermatitis herpetiformis, a **maternal uncle had reported similar symptoms.**

PE   Pallor.

Labs   CBC/PBS: **anemia;** reticulocyte count increased; megaloblastic cells, bite cells, and **Heinz bodies.** Serum indirect bilirubin increased. UA: positive for hemosiderin, methemalbumin, and hemoglobin; **G6PD enzyme assay normal (since the cells low in G6PD have already hemolyzed).** Six weeks later, G6PD enzyme assay is low.

Imaging   N/A

Gross Pathology   N/A

Micro Pathology   N/A

Treatment   Avoidance of drugs that may produce hemolysis. Circulatory support, maintenance of good renal blood flow, and transfusions with erythrocytes that are not G6PD deficient.

Discussion   G6PD is the first enzyme in the hexose monophosphate shunt. It **catalyzes the conversion of NADP+ to NADPH,** a powerful reducing agent. NADPH is a cofactor for glutathione reductase and thus plays a role in protecting the cell against oxidative attack. Ten percent of African-American males are affected, as are large numbers of black Africans and some inhabitants of Mediterranean areas. The disorder confers some selective advantage against endemic malaria. The gene for G6PD is on the **X chromosome** at band q28, and the pattern of inheritance is X-linked recessive.

. . . .

GLUCOSE-6-PHOSPHATE DEHYDROGENASE DEFICIENCY

ID/CC	A 50-year-old **Caucasian** male presents with progressively increasing **yellowing of the eyes** (= JAUNDICE), a peculiar **skin rash**, and **palpitations**.
HPI	On directed questioning, he admits to having **decreased libido**. Three years ago he was diagnosed with **diabetes** and is on oral hypoglycemics. He smokes and drinks alcohol only occasionally, has never received a blood transfusion, and has no prior history of jaundice.
PE	Generalized **bronze discoloration** of skin; irregularly irregular pulse; icterus; loss of pubic and axillary hair; testicular atrophy; gynecomastia; firm, nontender, nonpulsatile hepatomegaly.
Labs	Increased blood glucose; elevated LFTs; decreased serum testosterone and gonadotropins; **increased serum iron; decreased total iron-binding capacity; transferrin saturation > 80%; serum ferritin > 1000 µg/L (best screening method)**; desferrioxamine-chelatable urinary Fe excretion > 7.5 g Fe; **hepatic Fe quantitation > 100 µmol/g dry weight** (diagnostic). ECG: **atrial fibrillation**.
Imaging	CT-Abdomen: diffusely increased liver density. Echo: **dilated cardiomyopathy**.
Gross Pathology	Liver shows pigmentary cirrhosis.
Micro Pathology	Cirrhosis with abundant hemosiderin deposition in liver cells, Kupffer cells and bile ducts.
Treatment	Repeated phlebotomies; monitor for development of **hepatoma** (due to increased risk); **screening of first-degree relatives**.
Discussion	In idiopathic hemochromatosis, iron accumulates until the total body iron content reaches 50 g. The proximate cause is a breakdown in the normal control of iron absorption from the GI tract; normally, the amount of iron accumulated inversely affects the GI mucosal absorption of both heme and nonheme iron. As iron overload progresses, iron that is ordinarily stored in the cells of the reticuloendothelial system is deposited in the liver, joints, gonads, pancreas, heart, and skin. **FIRST AID** p.230

. . . .

HEMOCHROMATOSIS

ID/CC	A **10-year-old black child** presents with a chronic **nonhealing ulcer** on his lower leg.
HPI	He has had recurrent episodes of **abdominal and chest pain** (due to microvascular occlusion) along with **diminution of vision.** His maternal cousin suffers from a blood disorder.
PE	VS: fever. PS: **pallor; mild icterus;** funduscopy reveals **hypoxic spots with neovascularization** (= "SEA FANS"); nonhealing chronic ulcer on left lower leg.
Labs	CBC/PBS: decreased hematocrit; megaloblastic anemia; **sickle-shaped RBCs; Howell–Jolly bodies and Cabot rings; sickling of RBCs** on sodium metabisulfite peripheral film (Sickledex prep). Serum bilirubin moderately elevated; quantitative hemoglobin electrophoresis shows **85% HbS.** UA: microscopic hematuria.
Imaging	CT/ US-Abdomen: **small, calcified spleen.**
Gross Pathology	N/A
Micro Pathology	N/A
Treatment	Local therapy for leg ulcer; laser therapy for proliferative retinopathy; antibiotic prophylaxis against capsulated bacteria; **hydroxyurea** may help increase fetal hemoglobin levels.
Discussion	Caused by a **point mutation** on the gene coding for the beta chain of hemoglobin; shows **autosomal-recessive inheritance.** Glutamic acid is substituted by valine at position 6, leading to chronic hemolytic anemia. In the reduced form, HbS forms polymers that damage the RBC membrane. Factors that hasten sickling include acidosis and hypoxemia. Prenatal diagnosis is available for at-risk fetuses.

· ·

SICKLE CELL ANEMIA

ID/CC	A 30-year-old male is seen with complaints of **fever with chills, headache, and facial flushing immediately after a blood transfusion.**
HPI	He has aplastic anemia and received his **previous transfusion** a few weeks back. No such symptoms were reported during or immediately after that transfusion.
PE	VS: fever; tachycardia. PE: marked pallor; facial flushing; no cyanosis, icterus, or respiratory distress evident.
Labs	CBC: no leukocytosis; direct and indirect Coombs' test negative. Serum bilirubin normal; repeat **cross-matching** of donor serum and patient's blood reveals **no incompatibility.** UA: no hemoglobinuria.
Imaging	N/A
Gross Pathology	N/A
Micro Pathology	N/A
Treatment	Antipyretics, microaggregate factors to **filter out donor leukocytes** during future transfusions. Antihistamines, systemic steroids prior to transfusion.
Discussion	**Febrile reactions following transfusions are very common;** cytotoxic antibodies in the patient (developed following the previous transfusion) against the donor leukocytes produce a **type II hypersensitivity reaction.** Allergic reactions mediated by IgE result in an immediate type of hypersensitivity reaction directed against plasma proteins; mismatched blood transfusions result in hemolytic transfusion reactions.

. . . .

TRANSFUSION REACTION

ID/CC	A 60-year-old white female is seen with **insidious-onset forgetfulness and impairment of judgment,** with occasional acute episodes of **disorientation** with regard to time and place over the past three years.
HPI	She requires **frequent assistance** with daily activities and has had urinary incontinence over the past three months.
PE	Neurologic exam reveals marked disorientation with respect to time and place, mixed aphasia, and apraxia; pathologic mouth-opening responses; grasp reflex on right; and hyperactive responses in all four extremities.
Labs	Blood workup normal. LP: CSF normal. EEG: diffuse slowing of waves.
Imaging	CT: **brain atrophy resulting in enlargement of ventricular system and subarachnoid space.** PET: decreased glucose metabolism in parietal and temporal lobes.
Gross Pathology	Atrophic brain with narrow gyri and widened sulci; dilated lateral ventricles.
Micro Pathology	Postmortem findings include depletion of neurons, large neuritic plaques in cortex, **neurofibrillary tangles,** and eosinophilic inclusions in dendrites (= HIRANO BODIES).
Treatment	Supportive; tetrahydroaminoacridine (THAA).
Discussion	The most common cause of presenile dementia. Increased incidence in patients with Down's syndrome. FIRST AID p.233

ID/CC   A 28-year-old **woman** presents with a sudden, severe attack of vertigo associated with nausea and vomiting.

HPI   Her symptoms begin and are aggravated when she looks toward the right. She has no history of hearing loss, ear discharge, tinnitus, trauma, pain, or restricted neck movement.

PE   Symptoms recur when her head is turned toward right; rotatory fatigable nystagmus with a linear component; no hearing loss or any other neurologic deficit.

Labs   N/A

Imaging   N/A

Gross Pathology   N/A

Micro Pathology   N/A

Treatment   Reassurance and vestibular suppressants.

Discussion   The etiology of the condition is unknown but is sometimes seen after head injuries, ear operations, or infections of the middle ear; it may be due to degeneration of the statoconial membrane.

. . . .

BENIGN POSITIONAL VERTIGO

ID/CC	A 60-year-old male presents with **speech difficulties.**
HPI	The patient developed this difficulty following a **right-sided stroke** from which he is currently recovering. He is a **diabetic** who has been on insulin for 10 years, and he is also a **chronic smoker.**
PE	Speech **lacks fluency;** patient has difficulty **finding certain words** and sometimes **produces wrong word; comprehension is well preserved,** as are higher mental functions; ability to repeat is better than spontaneous speech; associated recovering right-sided aphasia noted; motor weakness of right upper and lower limbs with exaggerated deep tendon reflexes and right-sided Babinski's reflex.
Labs	Elevated blood glucose; remainder of tests normal.
Imaging	CT: **infarct in region of left frontoparietal cortex.**
Gross Pathology	N/A
Micro Pathology	N/A
Treatment	Speech **therapy** in addition to physiotherapy for stroke; long-term low-dose **aspirin.**
Discussion	Patient has Broca's dysphasia (expressive, nonfluent) with an associated right hemiplegia. The brain damage causing this condition is believed to involve the **dominant inferior frontal gyrus** (= BROCA'S AREA). **FIRST AID** p.235

. . . .

BROCA'S APHASIA

ID/CC	A 20-year-old male is brought to the ER after falling from a ladder.
HPI	He fell vertically so that his head hit the ground first. Despite the injury, he is conscious and **does not report any neurologic deficit,** only severe pain in his neck.
PE	**No neurologic deficit found** on clinical examination.
Labs	N/A
Imaging	XR-Cervical Spine: **burst fracture of atlas** (= JEFFERSON FRACTURE) with ring broken into four pieces.
Gross Pathology	N/A
Micro Pathology	N/A
Treatment	Inherently unstable fracture requiring halo jacket immobilization and fusion if nonunion occurs.
Discussion	The most common mechanism of injury in patients with Jefferson fracture is axial loading. Other cervical spine injuries include **atlantoaxial fracture dislocation,** more frequently associated with neurologic deficit; displacement is commonly anterior, and treatment consists of **skull traction** followed by **immobilization.** A **violent flexion–compression** force may result in a **sudden prolapse of the nucleus pulposus** of the cervical disc into the vertebral canal, producing quadriplegia; here an **early decompression** is required.

. . . .

C1 SPINAL CORD INJURY

ID/CC	A 70-year-old male presents with dull aching **pain in both calves after moderate exercise.**
HPI	The symptoms started a few months ago, typically developing after the patient walked 300–400 yards; **symptoms were relieved after a few minutes' rest or when the patient sat down and stooped forward.** In addition to the pain, the patient has experienced numbness in his thighs. He has had no sphincter disturbance but has had **low back pain for many years.**
PE	Spinal exam reveals **loss of lumbar lordosis** and reduced flexion and extension of lumbar spine; tone, power, and coordination in lower limbs normal; **reflexes in lower limbs symmetrical but reduced compared to upper limbs;** plantar reflexes flexor; peripheral arterial pulses **present** both at rest and after exercise.
Labs	Lab parameters normal.
Imaging	XR-Lumbar Spine: lumbar spondylosis with marked osteophyte formation. CT- Spine: **lumbar spinal canal stenosis confirmed.**
Gross Pathology	N/A
Micro Pathology	N/A
Treatment	Surgery requiring laminectomy at various levels.
Discussion	A number of mechanisms may lead to lumbar canal stenosis, including osteoarthritis with hypertrophy of the facet joints, disc prolapse, surgery, spondylolisthesis, Paget's disease, neoplasia, and infection; any of these conditions may be superimposed on a congenitally narrow spinal canal. The anteroposterior diameter of the cord is narrowed during extension, which tends to compromise the blood supply of the cord, resulting in the development of symptoms; stooping forward does the reverse and therefore relieves symptoms.

. . . .

CAUDA EQUINA SYNDROME

ID/CC	A 50-year-old male presents to the emergency room with **wild, flinging movements of his left arm and leg.**
HPI	He has been diagnosed with **diabetes and hypertension** but has taken his medications only irregularly. He is also a **chronic smoker.**
PE	Uncontrolled, violent, rapid flinging movements of left arm and leg; remainder of neurologic exam normal.
Labs	Lab tests reveal elevated blood glucose.
Imaging	CT (done at 48 hours): infarct in right **subthalamic nucleus.**
Gross Pathology	N/A
Micro Pathology	N/A
Treatment	Phenothiazines and dopamine agonists such as sulpiride and tetrabenazine may be of help.
Discussion	Hemiballismus is characterized by forceful, flinging, and violent movements, primarily of the proximal parts of the limbs of one side of the body, that disappear during sleep. The most common etiology is that of a vascular event in the contralateral subthalamic nucleus; other causes include an expanding arteriovenous malformation, trauma, tumor, and multiple sclerosis. Surgery may be indicated in cases of intractable involuntary movements.

ID/CC	A 56-year-old male with yellowing of the eyes and skin (due to **severe jaundice**) is brought to the ER in an **agitated state**.
HPI	He has been passing black, tarry, foul-smelling stools (= MELENA) and has exhibited a **reversal of sleep pattern** with **daytime sleepiness**. A few months ago he **vomited blood** (= HEMATEMESIS) and was admitted to the hospital, at which time he was diagnosed with **alcoholic liver cirrhosis.**
PE	VS: tachycardia; tachypnea; hypotension. PE: **lethargic and somnolent**; marked **icterus; feculent, fruity breath** (= FETOR HEPATICUS); signs of chronic liver disease found; asterixis, dysarthria, and primitive reflexes (suck and snout) demonstrated; exaggerated deep tendon reflexes; **ascites; liver span reduced; splenomegaly.**
Labs	LFTs markedly elevated (increased serum bilirubin, AST, and ALT; decreased serum albumin, reversed albumin-to-globulin ratio); alkaline phosphatase moderately elevated; prolonged PT; EEG: symmetric slowing; triphasic waves.
Imaging	Endoscopy (during previous admission): **bleeding esophageal varices.**
Gross Pathology	N/A
Micro Pathology	N/A
Treatment	**Eliminate precipitating factors**; institute high-calorie and very low-protein **diet; bowel cleansing** with **enemas; neomycin** and **lactulose** (induces diarrhea and clears the gut; alters bowel flora; and converts NH_3 to NH_4^+, which is less absorbable).
Discussion	The cause of hepatic encephalopathy is multifactorial and includes **elevated concentrations of blood ammonia, short-chain fatty acids, false neurotransmitters,** decreased branched-chain amino acids, and a circulating substance that has properties similar to that of benzodiazepine agonists that potentiate the action of **GABA.** **FIRST AID** p.249

· ·

HEPATIC ENCEPHALOPATHY

ID/CC	A **42-year-old** male presents with **depression,** poor memory, and **jerking movements** of the limbs and fingers.
HPI	His **father died of a similar** condition whose symptoms progressively worsened, proceeding to dementia until his death at the age of 50.
PE	**Chorea;** psychiatric evaluation reveals **cognitive impairment** (inattention and poor concentration without memory loss) and depression; no other focal neurologic deficit found.
Labs	Routine laboratory tests unremarkable.
Imaging	MR-Brain: degeneration of **caudate nucleus.** CT-Brain: cerebral atrophy.
Gross Pathology	Loss of brain mass with striking **atrophy of caudate nucleus** and, less strikingly, putamen; secondary loss of neurons in globus pallidus; cortical atrophy most commonly occurs in frontal lobe.
Micro Pathology	Degeneration of spiny GABAergic neurons in the striatum leads to a net loss of inhibitory signals from the striatum.
Treatment	No specific treatment available; supportive and symptomatic treatment.
Discussion	An autosomal-dominant disease whose gene locus is on chromosome 4, it is caused by expansion of a **trinucleotide repeat** (CAG) within the Huntington gene; expansion of the trinucleotide repeat leads to greater frequency of disease in successive generations (= GENETIC ANTICIPATION).

. . . .

HUNTINGTON'S CHOREA

ID/CC	A 25-year-old male is brought to a neurologist with complaints of **inability to see on one side.**
HPI	Two months ago he suffered **right eye optic neuritis,** but his vision has significantly improved since then, although it is not completely normal.
PE	On lateral gaze in either direction, one eye does not adduct and the other has **nystagmus** on abduction (finding characteristic of bilateral internuclear ophthalmoplegia); funduscopy reveals temporal pallor of right disc (due to atrophy of papillomacular fibers); visual field testing reveals right paracentral scotoma; **flexion of neck produces an electrical sensation that runs down back and into legs** (= LHERMITTE'S SIGN; suggests intramedullary disease of cervical cord).
Labs	LP: specific increase in CSF IgG concentration. Agarose electrophoresis reveals oligoclonal bands in IgG region of CSF. Evoked-potential studies of visual, auditory, and somatosensory pathways indicates impaired responses.
Imaging	MR- Brain (T2W): investigation of choice, **multiple, discreet, white-matter plaques.**
Gross Pathology	Sharply defined areas of gray discoloration (= PLAQUES) of white matter that occur particularly frequently around the ventricles and in the corpus callosum.
Micro Pathology	Active plaques show evidence of myelin breakdown, lipid-laden macrophages, and relative preservation of axons; lymphocytes and mononuclear cells prominent at edges of plaques.
Treatment	Immunosuppression (corticosteroids, azathioprine, cyclosporine), but success has been modest.
Discussion	The following are suggestive of multiple sclerosis: (1) Optic neuritis- early signs include diminished visual acuity, central or paracentral scotoma, hyperemia and edema of the optic disk, and a defective pupillary reaction to light. (2) Internuclear ophthalmoplegia (due to demyelination of the medial longitudinal fasciculus). (3) Lhermitte's sign.

. . . .

INTERNUCLEAR OPHTHALMOPLEGIA

ID/CC	A 15-year-old male is brought to a physician by his parents for an evaluation of recently observed **overindulgence in sexual activities.**
HPI	The parents also report that the patient's behavior has recently changed markedly from **aggressive to extremely placid;** directed questioning reveals that he has now started **exploring things orally** and has developed a voracious appetite. He suffered from **herpes simplex encephalitis** a few months ago. There is no history of prior psychiatric illness in the patient or in the family.
PE	Patient is in excellent health and is apparently unconcerned about his illness, displaying no reaction to parents' complaints; when physician attempts to shake his hand, patient begins to orally explore it; on seeing a nurse in doctor's room, he starts to masturbate.
Labs	N/A
Imaging	MR/ CT-Head: **bilateral temporal lobe and amygdala damage.**
Gross Pathology	N/A
Micro Pathology	N/A
Treatment	No specific treatment available.
Discussion	A syndrome of **hyperphagia, hypersexuality, placidity, and hyperorality.** In experimental animals, it results from **bilateral removal of the amygdala;** in humans, an incomplete picture is generally seen secondary to extensive temporal lobe damage, as may occur during herpes simplex encephalitis or in degenerative or post-traumatic brain damage.

. . . .

KLÜVER–BUCY SYNDROME

ID/CC   A 30-year-old female complains of **hoarseness, right shoulder drop, and difficulty turning her head to the left against resistance.**

HPI   Her mother suffers from neurofibromatosis.

PE   Absent gag reflex on right side; impaired taste sensation on posterior third of the tongue on right side; palatal movements reduced on right side and uvula deviated to left; right sternocleidomastoid is wasted and there is weakness in turning head toward left; shoulder is flattened and there is weakness of elevation of right shoulder (**lesion affecting CN IX, X, and XI**); tongue is normal (CN XII); no other neurologic deficits found.

Labs   N/A

Imaging   MR: mass, most likely a **neurofibroma** at base of skull around **region of jugular foramen.**

Gross Pathology   N/A

Micro Pathology   N/A

Treatment   Surgical removal if considered amenable to surgery.

Discussion   Causes of jugular foramen syndrome include neurofibroma of CN IX, X, or XI, meningiomas, cholesteatomas, glomus or carotid body tumors, metastases, granulomatous meningitis, and infection from the ear spreading into the posterior fossa.

ID/CC	A 60-year-old **woman** is seen with complaints of having difficulty walking and two episodes of **involuntary hand jerking** (= PARTIAL SEIZURE).
HPI	Her attendant reveals that over the past few months her **memory has deteriorated.** She has slow mentation and **urinary incontinence.** She is not diabetic or hypertensive.
PE	Funduscopy reveals papilledema; tone of lower limbs increased and strength reduced (= SPASTIC PARAPARESIS); deep tendon reflexes exaggerated; bilateral Babinski.
Labs	Routine laboratory tests normal.
Imaging	XR-Skull: **hyperostosis** of left parietal bone and sagittal suture. CT (with contrast): left parietal **parasagittal tumor.** MR (gadolinium): **intense tumor enhancement; dural extension** and invasion into superior sagittal sinus.
Gross Pathology	Irregular, firm, **gritty mass arising superficially, indenting and compressing brain but not invading it.**
Micro Pathology	**Whorling pattern** of meningothelial cells with regular, oval nuclei, indistinct cytoplasm, and **psammoma bodies.**
Treatment	Surgical resection. Radiation for unresectable cases.
Discussion	Primary intracranial neoplasm arising from cells of the **arachnoid granulations;** characterized by **slow growth, benign behavior, and expansile rather than infiltrative growth.** Common sites involved include the cerebral convexity, parasagittal (as in this case), sphenoid wing, olfactory groove, cerebellopontine angle, foramen magnum, and spinal cord. Tumor is usually solitary, is more common in women, and is found in middle and later ages.

. . . .

MENINGIOMA

ID/CC A 20-year-old woman complains of recurrent headaches associated with profound nausea and light sensitivity.

HPI She has had similar headaches several times each year since the onset of her menstrual periods. The headaches occur on one side of her head. She also reports seeing "flashing lights" like lightning moving across her field of vision. Stress, sleeplessness, and anxiety usually precipitate these headaches.

PE VS: normal. PE: funduscopic exam and visual field testing normal; neurologic exam normal.

Labs N/A

Imaging N/A

Gross Pathology N/A

Micro Pathology N/A

Treatment Prophylactic therapy with avoidance of precipitating factors and drugs such as beta-blockers, tricyclic antidepressants, or calcium channel blockers; abortive therapy during acute attacks with NSAIDs, sumatriptan, ergotamine, or transnasal butorphanol.

Discussion Migraine headache is the second most common cause of primary headache (the most common in the U.S. is tension headache). In the United States, an estimated 17% of women and 6% of men are affected by this disorder. The headache is characteristically preceded by a prodrome and is episodic, gradual in onset, usually unilateral, and most commonly in the temporal area. Its cause is unknown but appears to involve variations in cerebral blood flow and serotonergic pathways.

· ·

MIGRAINE

ID/CC	A **5-year-old male** is referred to a specialist by his physician for evaluation of an **abdominal mass** and a recently noticed **left-sided orbital proptosis.**
HPI	His parents complain of weight loss, poor feeding, and a continuous low-grade fever for the past few months.
PE	PE: marked **cachexia;** left-sided orbital proptosis and ecchymoses; large **intra-abdominal mass palpable.**
Labs	Marked **elevation of urinary catecholamines** and metabolites vanillylmandelic acid (VMA) and homovanillic acid (HVA).
Imaging	CT-Abdomen: **intra-abdominal mass arising from and obliterating left adrenal gland.** Nuc (bone scan): metastatic lytic lesion in left orbital region of skull.
Gross Pathology	Solid, round soft tumor mass obliterating left adrenal gland; **gray on cut surface** showing extensive hemorrhage and necrosis with cyst formation.
Micro Pathology	Anaplastic, small, round-to-oval hyperchromatic cells with scant cytoplasm in sheets and at places forming **Homer–Wright pseudorosettes;** few ganglion cells seen; electron microscopy reveals presence of **neurosecretory granules.**
Treatment	Surgical resection; chemotherapy with cyclophosphamide and adriamycin.
Discussion	A primary malignant neoplasm that arises from immature cells of the adrenal medulla and secretes catecholamines, it usually occurs in children under the age of five and presents with an abdominal mass. Hutchinson's neuroblastoma presents with extensive skull and orbital metastases that produce exophthalmos; metastases are common to lymph nodes, liver, lung, and bone.

. . . .

NEUROBLASTOMA

ID/CC	A 60-year-old male is seen by a neurologist for an evaluation of **deteriorating cognitive skills.**
HPI	Over the past few weeks, the patient has stayed in bed and has been incontinent with regard to both urine and feces.
PE	Cognition impaired; impaired ambulation without evidence of primary motor, sensory, or cerebellar dysfunction (= GAIT APRAXIA); deep tendon reflexes intact; pupils equal, round, and reactive to light and accommodation; plantars bilaterally flexor; fundus does not reveal any papilledema.
Labs	Lab parameters within normal limits.
Imaging	CT: **ventricular enlargement with relatively little cortical atrophy.** Nuc-Cisternography: persistent activity of radionuclide in lateral ventricles after 48 hours **(characteristic of normal pressure hydrocephalus).**
Gross Pathology	N/A
Micro Pathology	N/A
Treatment	Insertion of a ventriculoperitoneal shunt.
Discussion	In most patients, the cause of normal pressure hydrocephalus is not known, although it may follow a subarachnoid hemorrhage or meningitis (sometimes years later). The value of its early diagnosis lies in the fact that it is a **treatable dementia.**

ID/CC	A 35-year-old male who has been diagnosed with **multiple sclerosis** visits his physician with complaints of **difficulty swallowing** (= DYSPHAGIA) and **nasal regurgitation** of food.
HPI	Six months ago he suffered an attack of retrobulbar neuritis; two months ago he developed **spastic weakness of both lower limbs.**
PE	Speech is monotonous, slurred, and high-pitched (= "DONALD DUCK" DYSARTHRIA); dribbles from mouth; cannot protrude his **tongue, which lies on the floor of the mouth and is small and spastic;** palatal movements absent; jaw jerk exaggerated; patient is emotionally labile.
Labs	N/A
Imaging	MR- Brain: multiple focal white-matter plaques.
Gross Pathology	N/A
Micro Pathology	N/A
Treatment	General management of multiple sclerosis; no specific treatment available.
Discussion	The common causes of pseudobulbar palsy include bilateral cerebrovascular accidents involving the **internal capsule,** motor neuron disease, and multiple sclerosis.

ID/CC	A 50-year-old **man** is brought to the hospital by his neighbor in a **confused, drowsy state.**
HPI	He is a **chronic alcoholic** who has been drinking very heavily since his wife died and his sons deserted him. He has also become **unsteady in his gait and has often complained of numbness in his feet.**
PE	**Short-term memory poor and erratic;** on exam, patient produced details that appeared **unlikely to be true** on basis of his history (= CONFABULATIONS); fundi normal; evidence of **bilateral lateral rectus palsy** noted (bilateral VI nerve palsy); vertical **nystagmus** on upward gaze; **tongue and limbs tremulous;** bilateral **limb ataxia;** deep tendon reflexes present; plantars bilaterally flexor.
Labs	CBC: **megaloblastic anemia** (due to folate deficiency in alcoholics).
Imaging	CT-Head: thalamic and brainstem hemorrhages; enlarged cortical sulci and some evidence of cerebellar atrophy. MR: **mamillary body atrophy.**
Gross Pathology	Mamillary body atrophy.
Micro Pathology	Pathologically, Wernicke's encephalopathy is characterized by **atrophy of the mamillary bodies,** neuronal loss, and gliosis in the diencephalon and brainstem.
Treatment	Thiamine replacement therapy; abstinence from alcohol.
Discussion	Thiamine deficiency may cause Wernicke's encephalopathy, a disorder that usually occurs in alcoholics; the complete syndrome has classically been described as a triad of obtundation, ophthalmoplegia, and ataxia. Korsakoff's psychosis is characterized by anterograde and retrograde amnesia. Confabulation is often (but not invariably) present. **FIRST AID** p.235

. . . .

WERNICKE'S ENCEPHALOPATHY

ID/CC	A 16-year-old girl is seen with complaints of **colicky lower abdominal pain** together with nausea and vomiting associated with the **onset of menses.**
HPI	She achieved menarche at 14, and her initial cycles were irregular but painless (due to anovulation). She does not complain of any irregularity or excessive bleeding and has no urinary complaints or diarrhea.
PE	Abdominal exam normal; gynecologic exam reveals blood-stained pad; pelvic exam not performed due to intact hymen; rectal exam normal.
Labs	Routine lab parameters normal.
Imaging	N/A
Gross Pathology	N/A
Micro Pathology	N/A
Treatment	Symptomatic relief with **prostaglandin synthetase inhibitors** such as mefenamic acid or naproxen sodium; intractable symptoms may require **suppression of ovulation** using combined estrogen/progesterone or progestogens.
Discussion	**Primary dysmenorrhea** is defined as **painful periods** for which no organic or psychological cause can be found; the pain is colicky and usually begins shortly after or at the onset of menses. It is thought to be due to an increase in the production of prostaglandins and occurs **only during ovulatory cycles.**

. . . .

DYSMENORRHEA

ID/CC	A 32-year-old woman presents with **painful bilateral breast masses.**
HPI	The **pain is cyclic** in nature and **increases in her premenstrual phase**, at which time the **masses enlarge rapidly and then shrink.** She feels that both breasts are nodular and is concerned that she may have cancer.
PE	Mildly tender mass palpable in upper and outer quadrant of right and left breast; both **breasts nodular with multiple thickened areas;** no changes in overlying skin or nipple noted (vs. breast cancer); no axillary lymphadenopathy found.
Labs	Aspiration from breast mass reveals nonbloody fluid; **mass disappears completely after aspiration.**
Imaging	Mammo: nodularity and benign calcifications, no malignant features.
Gross Pathology	Cysts of various sizes ranging from microscopic to several millimeters surrounded by dense fibrotic tissue; contains clear or brown fluid.
Micro Pathology	Proliferation of acini in lobules (= SCLEROSING ADENOSIS).
Treatment	Reassurance and symptomatic management.
Discussion	Common in women between the ages of 35 and 55. Increased risk of invasive breast cancer in patients with epithelial hyperplasia and atypia.

FIBROCYSTIC DISEASE OF THE BREAST

ID/CC   A 30-year-old man complains of a small **painless nodular swelling over his right testicle** that he noticed a few months ago, coupled with **increasing growth of his breast tissue**.

HPI   He also complains of mild shortness of breath on exertion (= DYSPNEA), cough, and blood-streaked sputum.

PE   VS: normal. PE: bilateral gynecomastia (breast tissue palpable); small, **pea-shaped swelling** involving the **right testicle**; testicular sensation lost; no transillumination; **left supraclavicular lymphadenopathy**; hepatomegaly.

Labs   CBC: mild anemia. Serum **beta-hCG elevated**.

Imaging   CXR: two "cannonball" parenchymal masses (due to metastases). CT-Abdomen: enlarged retroperitoneal lymph nodes and multiple hepatic metastases. US-Scrotum: complex, solid right testicular mass.

Gross Pathology   Small, pea-shaped hemorrhagic mass seen in right testicle.

Micro Pathology   Polygonal, comparatively uniform **cytotrophoblastic cells** with clear cytoplasm growing in sheets and cords, mixed with **multinucleate syncytiotrophoblastic cells** that have **eosinophilic vacuolated cytoplasm** with readily **demonstrable hCG**; no well-developed villi seen.

Treatment   **Chemotherapy** with **cisplatin, methotrexate, and bleomycin** in some combination, followed by **radical inguinal orchiectomy** and **retroperitoneal lymph node dissection**; gynecomastia regresses once the source of hCG (the tumor) is removed.

Discussion   **Choriocarcinoma** is the **most malignant** of all testicular tumors; it metastasizes relatively early via both the **lymphatics** and the **bloodstream** even when it remains locally very small. **Follow up with beta-hCG levels.**

. . . .

GYNECOMASTIA WITH TESTICULAR CHORIOCARCINOMA

ID/CC	A 55-year-old woman presents with a **painless left breast lump** that she discovered on self-examination.
HPI	N/A
PE	**Fixed, 2-cm, indurated, nontender mass palpable** in upper and outer quadrant of left breast; **dimpling** of skin above left nipple seen when patient raises left hand above head; painless left axillary **lymphadenopathy**.
Labs	N/A
Imaging	Mammo: dense spiculated mass with pleomorphic calcifications.
Gross Pathology	N/A
Micro Pathology	Trucut needle biopsy shows **neoplastic cells streaming through desmoplastic stroma;** one duct is filled with malignant cells displaying a **cribriform** pattern.
Treatment	Modified radical mastectomy, adjuvant chemotherapy and radiotherapy if required.
Discussion	**Most common type of breast cancer;** occurs as an irregular, unilateral, hard nodule averaging 1–2 cm in size. These tumors are graded according to the **degree of nuclear atypia** and **histologic** (tubule) **differentiation**.

· ·

INFILTRATING DUCTAL CARCINOMA

ID/CC	A **70-year-old woman** presents with a **painful enlargement** of her left breast.
HPI	Two years ago she underwent a **right mastectomy for an infiltrating ductal carcinoma.**
PE	Left breast **warm and edematous** and has **swollen red** discoloration with **peau d'orange** appearance involving more than half of the breast; diffusely indurated and tender on palpation; **axillary lymphadenopathy** noted.
Labs	N/A
Imaging	Mammo: **diffusely increased density** in the left breast with skin thickening.
Gross Pathology	N/A
Micro Pathology	Biopsy reveals large spheroidal cells and fine stroma **infiltrated by lymphocytes.**
Treatment	Chemotherapy is treatment employed; outcome is universally fatal.
Discussion	**Previous breast cancer is a risk factor** for cancer in the contralateral breast. This is the **most malignant** form of breast cancer and implies angiolymphatic spread.

. . . .

INFLAMMATORY CARCINOMA OF BREAST

ID/CC	A 46-year-old **woman** presents with a palpable mass in the left breast.
HPI	The patient has been admitted to the hospital to obtain an excisional biopsy and for planning further management. The **patient's older sister recently died of metastatic breast cancer.**
PE	Left breast mass on palpation; nipples normally located without evidence of retraction; no evidence of axillary lymphadenopathy or hepatomegaly.
Labs	N/A
Imaging	Mammo: frequently normal or an asymmetric density without definable margins.
Gross Pathology	Firm, white, irregularly shaped 3 cm mass was removed from each breast.
Micro Pathology	Histologic sections reveal terminal lobules distended by intermediate-sized cells with scant mitotic activity; neoplastic cells infiltrate the stroma with individual neoplastic cells in a single file (= INDIAN FILE PATTERN) that surrounds the terminal lobule in a target-appearing fashion.
Treatment	Modified radical mastectomy with axillary lymph node sampling; adjuvant chemotherapy and radiotherapy if required. Frequent mammographic surveillance due to high incidence of second primary in same or opposite breast.
Discussion	Infiltrating lobular carcinoma is the most common malignancy of the terminal lobule. It accounts for 10% – 13% of all breast cancers.

LOBULAR CARCINOMA OF THE BREAST

ID/CC	A 25-year-old **woman** complains of **loss of weight** and intense right lower abdominal pain and nausea that began when she went jogging yesterday afternoon.
HPI	Intermittent episodes of similar pain have occurred over the past several days. She has regular menstrual cycles with average flow and no dysmenorrhea and had her last period three weeks ago.
PE	VS: mild hypotension; normal HR (HR 90). PE: **right lower quadrant tenderness**; pelvic exam: tender 6-cm **right adnexal mass** anterior to uterus.
Labs	CBC: normal; pregnancy test negative.
Imaging	XR-KUB: irregular **calcified** mass in region of right ovary. US-Pelvis: **cystic tumor** about 8 cm in diameter replacing the right ovary.
Gross Pathology	Cystic mass replacing the right ovary; thin, **fibrous wall with solid nodule at one aspect containing sebaceous material and matted hair**; tooth structures also seen.
Micro Pathology	Mature tissue elements **representing all three germ cell layers** are present, including skin with adnexal structures, bone, cartilage, teeth, thyroid, bronchi, intestine, and neural tissue.
Treatment	Surgical resection curative.
Discussion	Primary benign teratomas or dermoid cysts originate from germ cells; tumors are cystic and contain elements of all three germ cell layers. Complications of teratomas include torsion, infection, rupture leading to chemical peritonitis, infertility, secretion of thyroid hormone leading to hyperthyroidism (= STRUMA OVARII), and carcinoid syndrome due to serotonin secretion; rarely, squamous cell carcinoma may develop in a dermoid cyst.

OVARIAN TERATOMA

ID/CC	A **23-year-old** married **woman** is seen with complaints of **inability to conceive** after a year of unprotected intercourse (= INFERTILITY).
HPI	Her last menstrual period was three months ago, and since menarche she **has only 4–5 periods each year** (= OLIGOMENORRHEA); a pregnancy test at home was negative. She also complains of **excessive facial hair.** Her **father was diabetic.**
PE	Patient **obese;** excessive **facial hair and male-pattern hair distribution on rest of body** (= HIRSUTISM) but no virilization; pelvic exam normal; secondary sexual characteristics well developed.
Labs	**Elevated LH; decreased FSH** and loss of normal periodicity (LH > FSH, 3:1 ratio); **serum testosterone and androstenedione elevated; serum estradiol** (total and free) within normal limits in early and midfollicular phases; **pattern of secretion abnormal with no preovulatory or midluteal increase;** TSH and prolactin levels normal.
Imaging	US-Transvaginal (high resolution): morphologic features of **polycystic ovaries** (multiple peripheral follicles < 8 mm in diameter; prominent echodense stroma).
Gross Pathology	Ovaries enlarged with **pearly white capsule** and multiple cysts averaging 1 cm in diameter within stroma.
Micro Pathology	Cysts **lined by granulosa and theca cells,** the latter luteinized; stroma shows **hyperthecosis** and fibrosis.
Treatment	Reduce weight; ovulation induction with clomiphene; laparoscopic ovarian diathermy or laser drilling in drug-resistant cases; low-dose combined contraceptive pill if contraception is desired.
Discussion	Polycystic ovarian syndrome (**Stein–Leventhal Syndrome**) is a clinical syndrome of **obesity, hirsutism, and secondary amenorrhea or oligomenorrhea with infertility due to anovulation,** accompanied by multiple-follicle cysts within both ovaries. PCOS patients are at increased risk for breast and endometrial carcinomas (due to unopposed LH stimulation).

. . . .

POLYCYSTIC OVARY DISEASE

ID/CC	A 38-year-old **grand multipara** develops a marked drop in her blood pressure following **uncontrolled bleeding immediately after delivery.**
HPI	She delivered **twins** at 35 weeks' gestation with **polyhydramnios.**
PE	VS: **hypotension; tachycardia.** PE: anxious; pallor; low central venous pressure; **uterus soft and flabby** with indistinct outline.
Labs	CBC: anemia; mildly decreased hematocrit. Coagulation profile normal.
Imaging	N/A
Gross Pathology	Uterus **grossly overdistended and flabby.**
Micro Pathology	N/A
Treatment	**Fluid resuscitation; blood transfusion;** rub up a **uterine contraction;** maintain contraction with an oxytocin infusion; if found, **remove retained placenta;** check for cervical, vaginal, or uterine lacerations and uterine rupture; hypogastric artery ligation and/or hysterectomy if other measures fail.
Discussion	Primary postpartum hemorrhage (PPH) is defined as loss of 500 mL or more of blood within 24 hours of delivery, or any amount of bleeding that is sufficient to produce a hemodynamic compromise; primary causes include uterine atony, retained placenta, and soft tissue injury. Factors associated with an increased risk of uterine atony and retained placenta include **high multiparity, a maternal age > 35 years, delivery after an antepartum hemorrhage, multiple pregnancies, polyhydramnios, a past history of PPH, and coagulation disorders.** Sheehan's syndrome—a clinical syndrome of hypopituitarism secondary to ischemic pituitary necrosis—is a peculiar complication of massive postpartum hemorrhage.

. . . .

ID/CC	A 65-year-old **nulliparous woman** is referred for intractable vulval **pruritus** and a vulvar growth.
HPI	She has also felt an obstruction in the flow of her urine. She was a **prostitute** and was treated often for STDs. She is a **chronic smoker.**
PE	Gynecologic exam reveals excoriation marks over vulva; exophytic growth arising from left labia majora; left inguinal lymphadenopathy.
Labs	Cystoscopy reveals lower urethral stenosis (due to involvement by vulval growth).
Imaging	N/A
Gross Pathology	Gross exam: exophytic growth.
Micro Pathology	Microscopic exam of punch biopsy specimen reveals invasive, well-differentiated **squamous cell carcinoma with keratinization.**
Treatment	Confirm diagnosis; preoperative radiotherapy to shrink tumor mass; radical vulvectomy with lymph node dissection.
Discussion	Vulvar cancer is a disease of **older women** with a mean age of 60 years. It is associated with **nulliparity** and **smoking,** and its recent increase in incidence among younger women is associated with **papillomavirus.** Carcinoma in situ (vulval intraepithelial neoplasia, or VIN) and squamous dysplasia are considered precursor lesions.

. . . .

VULVAR CARCINOMA

ID/CC	A 45-year-old male is seen with complaints of **blurring of vision while reading and performing similar tasks involving near vision.**
HPI	He complains that he has to hold the newspaper at an increasing distance in order to read it clearly. He has had no previous problems with his vision and has no history of diabetes or hypertension.
PE	**Amplitude of accommodation reduced;** convex lens reduced near-point distance, allowing patient to read comfortably and to engage in tasks requiring near vision.
Labs	N/A
Imaging	N/A
Gross Pathology	N/A
Micro Pathology	N/A
Treatment	Convex lens glasses for work requiring near vision.
Discussion	**Natural loss of accommodation** (= PRESBYOPIA) due to **sclerosis of the lens substance,** which fails to adapt itself to a more spherical shape when the zonule is relaxed in the accommodation reflex.

ID/CC	A 29-year-old woman visits a clinic with complaints of **visual blurring**.
HPI	She also complains of **headaches** that are worse in the morning. She has been taking **oral contraceptives** for some time.
PE	VS: normotension. PE: patient is **obese;** funduscopy reveals presence of **papilledema;** no focal neurologic deficit noted; remainder of exam normal.
Labs	N/A
Imaging	CT: ventricles normal, increased volume of subarachnoid spaces. Angio: rules out dural sinus thrombosis.
Gross Pathology	N/A
Micro Pathology	N/A
Treatment	Stop oral contraceptives, advised diuretics and obesity-reducing measures.
Discussion	Benign intracranial hypertension is primarily a disease of **obese females;** its etiology is unknown, although associations exist with the use of certain drugs (oral contraceptives, steroids, nalidixic acid, tetracycline) as well as with pregnancy, previous head injury, dural sinus thrombosis, and excessive vitamin A intake.

ID/CC   A **16-year-old male** is referred to an ophthalmologist for an evaluation of a **progressively constricting visual field.**

HPI   The boy complains that he sees as though he were looking **through a narrow tube.** Directed questioning reveals that he has a long-standing history of **night blindness.** His parents, although normal, had a **consanguineous marriage** and have a **family history of a visual disorder.**

PE   Funduscopy reveals **"bone spicule" pigmentation** in mid-periphery of fundus, waxy appearance of optic disc, and marked narrowing and attenuation of vessels; **field of vision shows concentric contraction** that is especially marked if illumination is reduced.

Labs   Electroretinogram and electro-oculogram demonstrate reduced activity.

Imaging   N/A

Gross Pathology   N/A

Micro Pathology   N/A

Treatment   No satisfactory treatment; genetic counseling for prevention of the disease if the pattern of inheritance in a particular family can be traced.

Discussion   Retinitis pigmentosa is a slow degenerative disease of the retina that is always bilateral, begins in childhood, and results in blindness by middle or advanced age; the degeneration primarily affects the rods and the cones, particularly the cones, and commences in a zone near the equator, spreading both anteriorly and posteriorly. The condition may be associated with Laurence–Moon–Biedl syndrome (characterized by obesity, hypogenitalism, and mental subnormality), Refsum's disease (peripheral neuropathy, cerebellar ataxia, deafness, and ichthyosis due to a defect in phytanic acid metabolism), and abetalipoproteinemia. The condition is inherited as an autosomal-recessive trait in 40% of cases, as autosomal-dominant in 20%, and as X-linked in 5%.

. . . .

RETINITIS PIGMENTOSA

ID/CC	A 25-year-old female **athlete** is brought to the ER after she hurt her right knee.
HPI	She had **fallen on a hyperextended right knee** that has been unstable since the fall.
PE	Right knee: effusion and **positive anterior "draw sign"** (tibia can be pulled forward on femur with knee flexed); instability of right knee joint (demonstrated by moving upper end of tibia forward on femur with knee flexed only 10–20 degrees [= LACHMAN TEST]).
Labs	N/A
Imaging	MR- Knee: indistinct, heterogenous signal in expected region of the anterior cruciate ligament.
Gross Pathology	N/A
Micro Pathology	N/A
Treatment	Plaster cylinder for three weeks followed by hamstring and quadriceps exercises.
Discussion	The anterior cruciate ligament is torn by a force driving the upper end of the tibia forward relative to the femur or by hyperextension of the knee; the **posterior cruciate ligament is torn by a force driving the upper end of the tibia backward.**

. . . .

ANTERIOR CRUCIATE LIGAMENT INJURY

ID/CC A **60-year-old woman** is brought to the orthopedic clinic with complaints of **pain in the left hip and inability to bear weight** on the left leg.

HPI **Three years** ago she sustained a **fracture of the neck of the femur** that was treated with internal fixation. She is an **alcoholic** and has been taking **oral steroids** for many years for a chronic skin ailment.

PE All movements at left hip are restricted by pain; unable to bear weight on the limb.

Labs N/A

Imaging XR-Left Hip: **increase in bone density of femoral head** and collapse of articular surface; dynamic hip screw in place. MR-Hip: more sensitive.

Gross Pathology N/A

Micro Pathology N/A

Treatment **Total hip replacement arthroplasty** significantly reduces morbidity.

Discussion **Fracture of the neck of the femur is the most common cause** of avascular necrosis of the femoral head; other risk factors include excessive alcohol consumption, steroid therapy, radiation therapy, and deep sea diving (**Caisson's disease**). Normally **blood is supplied to the head by three routes:** through vessels in the ligamentum teres, through capsular vessels reflected onto the femoral neck, and through branches of nutrient vessels within the substance of the bone. When the fracture occurs, nutrient vessels are necessarily severed, capsular vessels are injured to varying degrees, and **blood supply is maintained only through the vessels in the ligamentum teres.** This is a variable quantity and is often insufficient, resulting in avascular necrosis of the femoral head.

. . . .

AVASCULAR NECROSIS OF THE FEMORAL HEAD

ID/CC	A 40-year-old woman presents with **numbness and an unpleasant tingling sensation** (= PARESTHESIA) **on the palmar side of her right thumb, the second and third fingers, and the radial side of her fourth finger.**
HPI	She suffers from **rheumatoid arthritis.**
PE	**Wasting of thenar eminence;** weakness while apposing thumb to fifth digit (weakness of opponens pollicis); tapping over transverse carpal ligament and forced flexion of wrists in downward direction reproduces symptoms.
Labs	N/A
Imaging	N/A
Gross Pathology	N/A
Micro Pathology	N/A
Treatment	**Decompression** of the tunnel by a longitudinal incision of the flexor retinaculum.
Discussion	This condition is seen in people who use their hands a lot. Other causes include rheumatoid arthritis, hypothyroidism, amyloidosis, and pregnancy.

· ·

CARPAL TUNNEL SYNDROME

ID/CC   A 55-year-old woman presents with an **aching pain in the back of her neck**, a feeling of stiffness, and a **"grating" sensation upon movement.**

HPI   She also has a history of a vague, ill-defined, and ill-localized pain spreading over her shoulder region. She does not complain of any noticeable motor weakness or sensory loss over any part of the body and has no bladder or bowel complaints.

PE   Neck **slightly kyphotic; posterior cervical muscles tender; neck movements** slightly **restricted at extremes** due to pain; **audible crepitation on movement; diminished supinator and biceps reflex in the left upper limb;** no motor or sensory loss demonstrable.

Labs   N/A

Imaging   XR-Cervical Spine (lateral view): **narrowing of intervertebral disc space with formation of osteophytes at vertebral margins,** especially anteriorly.

Gross Pathology   N/A

Micro Pathology   N/A

Treatment   There is a strong tendency for the **symptoms of cervical spondylosis to subside spontaneously.** Treatment includes **analgesics, physiotherapy, and support of the neck** by a closely fitting collar of plaster or plastic.

Discussion   Degenerative arthritis occurs predominantly in the **lowest three cervical joints.** The changes **first affect the central intervertebral joints and later affect the posterior intervertebral (facet) joints. Osteophytes commonly encroach on the intervertebral foramina,** reducing the space for transmission of the cervical nerves. If the restricted space is further reduced by the traumatic edema of the contained soft tissues, manifestations of nerve pressure are likely to occur. Rarely, the spinal cord itself may suffer damage, producing a cervical myelopathy.

. . . .

CERVICAL SPONDYLOSIS

ID/CC	A **14-year-old male** is admitted to the hospital complaining of **pain** and **swelling** in the left **leg.**
HPI	The pain has been present for two months but has become progressively worse over that period. There is no history of trauma or infection.
PE	VS: **mild fever.** PE: tenderness and fusiform swelling over left femur.
Labs	Elevated ESR. Karyotype: **translocation of the long arms of chromosomes 11 and 22.**
Imaging	XR-Left Femur: lytic lesion in medullary zone of midshaft with cortical destruction and **"onion-skin"** appearance. CXR: no evidence of metastatic spread.
Gross Pathology	Large areas of bone lysis as tumors erode cancellous trabeculae of long bones outward to cortex.
Micro Pathology	Biopsy of bone reveals sheets of uniform, small cells resembling lymphocytes; in many places tumor cells surround a central clear area, forming a **"pseudorosette."** **Cell origin of tumor is unknown.**
Treatment	**"Melt" tumor with radiotherapy;** surgical resection; regular follow-up for recurrence.
Discussion	**Diaphysis** of the long bones is the **most common site of occurrence** of Ewing's sarcoma. Five-year survival is only 10%, with the cause of death being widespread hematogenous dissemination.

· ·

EWING'S SARCOMA

ID/CC	A 40-year-old **laborer** is brought to the ER with sudden-onset **severe back pain after lifting a heavy object.**
HPI	The pain is made worse by **movement, coughing, and straining** and radiates to the right buttock and thigh. He also complains of **weakness and patchy loss of sensation in the right leg.** He reports no urinary or bowel incontinence.
PE	PE: tenderness at level of **L5–S1 vertebrae;** restricted straight leg raising (due to pain); loss of pain and temperature sensation over back of right thigh and buttock; weakness of right toe extensors (L5) and right foot evertors (S1); diminished right ankle jerk; anal sphincter tone normal.
Labs	N/A
Imaging	XR-Lumbar Spine: loss of lumbar lordosis and vertebral osteophytes. MR-Spine: posterolateral (right) **herniation producing nerve root compression at level of L5-S1.**
Gross Pathology	N/A
Micro Pathology	N/A
Treatment	Surgical laminectomy in this case due to muscle weakness arising out of nerve root compression.
Discussion	Degenerative changes in the annulus fibrosus and paraspinal ligaments lead to **herniation of the nucleus pulposus into the spinal canal;** minor trauma is usually sufficient to precipitate symptoms. The annulus fibrosus most commonly **protrudes or ruptures lateral to the posterior longitudinal ligament.** The herniation of disk material may compress one or more nerve roots, leading to radicular pain and to either sensory or motor deficits. Lumbar disk herniation **most commonly affects the S1 nerve root at the L5–S1 level or the L5 nerve root at the L4–L5 level.**

. . . .

HERNIATED DISC

ID/CC	A 20-year-old male is brought to the ER with complaints of pain and inability to use his left forearm.
HPI	He was hurt while trying to ward off an assault by a drunken roommate.
PE	PE: **unable to pronate and supinate left forearm; fracture in upper half of ulna.**
Labs	N/A
Imaging	XR-Left Forearm: fracture of upper half of ulna with dislocation of the radial head.
Gross Pathology	N/A
Micro Pathology	N/A
Treatment	Open reduction and plating followed by four weeks in plaster.
Discussion	This is a fracture of the **upper third of the ulna** with dislocation of the radial head caused by a fall on an outstretched hand, with the forearm forced into excessive pronation. It may also result from a direct blow on the back of the upper forearm.

. . . .

MONTEGGIA'S FRACTURE

ID/CC   A **30-year-old woman** is brought to the ER after a **minor fall** in which she sustained a **fracture** of her left lower leg.

HPI   She has a history of **pain in her limbs and joints.** She had been complaining of **increased thirst** (= POLYDIPSIA) and **increased urination** (= POLYURIA) and one month ago she was operated on for **multiple renal stones.** She also complains of **indigestion** and poorly localized **abdominal pain** and has been receiving treatment for endogenous **depression.**

PE   VS: hypertension. PE: anxious-looking; fracture of both bones of left lower leg.

Labs   **Increased serum calcium** (> 10.5 mg/dL); **decreased phosphate** (< 2.5 mg/dL); **increased serum PTH;** increased urinary phosphate.

Imaging   XR-Left Leg (AP and lateral views): fracture of tibia and fibula; **diffuse osteoporosis** with marked thinning of cortex and **scattered fibrocystic changes** (pathologically "brown cysts"). Other x-rays: rarefaction of the whole skeleton with marked loss of density and very thin cortices; scattered cystic changes in long bones, and skull showed uniform fine, granular mottling (= SALT AND PEPPER APPEARANCE) with small, translucent cystlike areas. XR-KUB: **nephrolithiasis** and **nephrocalcinosis.**

Gross Pathology   Surgical exploration: one of the parathyroid glands enlarged above normal.

Micro Pathology   Resected tissue: thinly encapsulated mass of **chief cells** compressing surrounding gland.

Treatment   Surgical resection of adenoma.

Discussion   Primary hyperparathyroidism is usually caused either by an adenoma or less commonly by primary hyperplasia or carcinoma; it may be sporadic or, in younger patients, may be familial and linked to multiple endocrine neoplasia (MEN) syndromes types I and IIa. Secondary hyperplasia may be produced by chronic renal failure.

· ·

OSTEITIS FIBROSA CYSTICA
(HYPERPARATHYROIDISM)

ID/CC	A 27-year-old male comes to the ER visits the emergency room due to a swollen right wrist.
HPI	A few minutes ago, he **sustained a fall on his outstretched right hand.**
PE	Right wrist swollen; **tenderness in anatomical snuff box** and on AP compression of scaphoid.
Labs	N/A
Imaging	XR-Right Wrist (oblique, AP, and lateral views): no fracture noted initially, but on repeating XRs **after two weeks,** a **fracture line** was seen at the waist of the right scaphoid. Nuc: increased uptake of scaphoid.
Gross Pathology	N/A
Micro Pathology	N/A
Treatment	Immobilize wrist in a knuckle-to-elbow plaster, including the thumb as far as the interphalangeal joint. Follow up with x-rays to confirm bone union and healing.
Discussion	Complications of the fracture **include avascular necrosis of the proximal segment** (blood supply to the bone goes from distal to proximal, and hence there is a risk of avascular necrosis of the proximal fragment), delayed union, and nonunion (the scaphoid spans both rows of carpal bones; hence the high risk of nonunion); if nonunion is associated with symptoms, bone grafting and internal fixation should be undertaken. Osteoarthritis of the wrist is a long-term sequela.

SCAPHOID FRACTURE

ID/CC	A 40-year-old male is brought to the ER after sustaining **a fall on his outstretched hand;** the patient supports the right arm, which is **abducted.**
HPI	The patient complains of pain and inability to move his shoulder.
PE	Right arm abducted; **normal contour of right shoulder joint lost and flattened;** fullness observed below clavicle that can be felt to move on rotating arm (due to displaced head); patient cannot touch his opposite shoulder; pain and temperature sensation lost on skin over acromion (due to **axillary nerve damage**).
Labs	N/A
Imaging	XR-Right Shoulder (AP view): humeral head lies well below glenoid fossa.
Gross Pathology	N/A
Micro Pathology	N/A
Treatment	Reduction under general anesthesia.
Discussion	The most common form is **anterior shoulder dislocation** and is caused by a fall on the outstretched hand; in younger patients, the capsule is strong and does not tear. The glenoid labrum and capsule are avulsed from the bone, allowing recurrent dislocations to occur. In older patients, the capsule is torn and heals after reduction. Recurrent dislocation is less common among older patients.

. . . .

SHOULDER DISLOCATION

ID/CC	A 12-year-old obese male is brought to the hospital with complaints of sudden-onset pain of the left hip and limp.
HPI	The pain is felt in the left groin and often radiates to the left thigh and knee.
PE	Left leg **externally rotated and about 2 cm shorter;** limited range of abduction and internal rotation; **upon flexing left hip, knee is drawn toward left axilla.**
Labs	N/A
Imaging	XR-Left Hip (AP view): **growth plate widened and irregular.**
Gross Pathology	N/A
Micro Pathology	N/A
Treatment	Head was fixed with pins or screws to prevent further slipping.
Discussion	Slipped femoral epiphyses affects youth **10–18 years old,** with boys more commonly affected than girls; affected children may be overweight and in some cases have delayed sexual development. Represents a Salter-Harris type I epiphyseal injury. Twenty-five percent are bilateral, of which 15%–20% occur simultaneously. **Avascular necrosis** of the femoral head and **osteoarthritis** may arise as complications.

ID/CC	A 35-year-old male seen after a roadside accident presents with a **persistent bloody but thin nasal discharge**.
HPI	Directed questioning reveals that he has also **lost his sense of smell** since the accident.
PE	Watery nasal discharge noted; **bilateral periorbital hematomas** ("black eye") seen; **anosmia** found on neurologic exam; remainder of physical exam normal; on placing a drop of nasal discharge on clean white gauze, **spreading yellow halo noted in addition to central blood stain** (= "HALO SIGN"; due to presence of CSF).
Labs	N/A
Imaging	CT-Head: **fracture of cribriform plate.**
Gross Pathology	N/A
Micro Pathology	N/A
Treatment	Antibiotics; head end elevated by 30 degrees; patient **advised not to blow his nose**; neurosurgical consult for possible repair of meninges.
Discussion	Fractures of the base of the skull involve the anterior or middle cranial fossa. Those affecting the anterior fossa, as in this case, may cause nasal bleeding, periorbital hematomas, subconjunctival hemorrhages, CSF rhinorrhea, and cranial nerve injuries (CN I–V); **middle cranial fossa structures involving the petrous temporal bone may cause bleeding from the ear, CSF otorrhea, bruising over the ear over the mastoid (= "BATTLE SIGN"), and cranial nerve injuries (CN VII–VIII).**

· ·

CRIBRIFORM PLATE FRACTURE

ID/CC	A 30-year-old male complains of sudden-onset **dizziness, nausea, vomiting (nonprojectile), and loss of balance.**
HPI	He also complains of headache and blurred vision (due to nystagmus). He has **chronic suppurative otitis media** (CSOM) of the right ear, for which he has taken treatment irregularly.
PE	Patient lying on left ear and looking toward right ear; **conductive deafness** (Rinne negative; Weber lateralized toward right ear) in right ear; horizontal spontaneous nystagmus toward left; purulent ear discharge from right ear; no neurologic deficits.
Labs	N/A
Imaging	XR-Mastoid Area: **obliteration of mastoid air cells on right side.**
Gross Pathology	N/A
Micro Pathology	N/A
Treatment	Surgical exploration of mastoid; antibiotics and vestibular suppressants.
Discussion	Pyogenic inflammation of the labyrinth may result from acute otitis media, operations on the stapes, or preformed pathways such as fracture lines; in CSOM, cholesteatoma may cause erosion of the semicircular canals, exposing the labyrinth to infections.

. . . .

LABYRINTHITIS

ID/CC A 40-year-old **man** complains that "the whole room seems to be spinning" (= VERTIGO) while also experiencing ringing in the ears (= TINNITUS) and nausea.

HPI The patient also complains of a **sense of fullness** in his ears and adds that his **hearing has progressively diminished** over the past few years. His symptoms were initially **unilateral but have now become bilateral.** His illness has run a course of **remissions and relapses.** He denies any weakness of the limbs and has no history of ear discharge or trauma.

PE VS: normal. PE: anxious; neurologic exam normal; caloric tests bilaterally normal.

Labs Pure-tone audiometry reveals **sensorineural hearing loss** that is more marked for **lower frequencies;** loudness recruitment present; short-increment sensitivity index (SISI) shows high score; VDRL negative.

Imaging MR/CT-Head: normal (performed to rule out internal auditory canal pathology).

Gross Pathology N/A

Micro Pathology **Gross distention of the endolymphatic system (=** ENDOLYMPHATIC HYDROPS).

Treatment No specific treatment; symptomatic relief with **vestibular suppressants and diuretics.** Surgical intervention is controversial.

Discussion A disease of the inner ear characterized by **acute onset** and **recurrent attacks of vertigo,** it is often associated with nausea and vomiting **together with diminished hearing and tinnitus.** Although the exact etiology is unknown, endolymphatic hydrops (due to excess of endolymph in the scala media) has been linked to obstruction of resorption, defective membrane exchange, and increased endolymph inflow (secondary to allergy, vasomotor factors, or retained sodium and water).

. . . .

MENIÈRE'S DISEASE

ID/CC	A 60-year-old male complains of **progressively diminishing hearing acuity over the past few years.**
HPI	The patient's hearing loss is **bilateral** and is almost the **same for both ears;** he has no history of ear discharge, tinnitus, or trauma.
PE	Ability to distinguish between consonants markedly impaired; **air conduction more than bone conduction** (due to sensorineural hearing loss); audiometry reveals **bilateral hearing loss in higher-frequency range.**
Labs	N/A
Imaging	N/A
Gross Pathology	N/A
Micro Pathology	Presbycusis is characterized by a loss of hair cells, atrophy of the spinal ganglion, altered endolymph production, and thickening of the basilar membrane with some neural degeneration.
Treatment	Counseling; some help could be obtained from a hearing aid.
Discussion	A type of sensorineural hearing loss that results from the **aging process;** degenerative changes occur in the cells of the organ of Corti and nerve fibers. Deafness is bilateral and symmetrical, commonly **affecting the high tones.** Other types of presbycusis include strial, which starts in the fourth and sixth decades, is slowly progressive, and is characterized by good discrimination and the presence of recruitment, a flat or descending audiogram, and patchy atrophy of the middle and apical turns of the stria. Cochlear deafness begins in middle age and is of the conductive variety, showing a downward slope on audiogram and absent pathologic findings. Both types of sensorineural loss can be avoided through use of protection in high-noise areas and monitoring of ototoxic drugs.

· ·

PRESBYCUSIS

ID/CC	A 50-year-old male complains of **hearing loss and a whistling sound in his left ear** (= TINNITUS).
HPI	He claims to have pronounced **difficulty understanding speech** (out of proportion to hearing loss). He has also experienced occasional **vertigo**.
PE	Left-sided **sensorineural deafness**; Weber test lateralized **toward right ear**; left-sided corneal reflex lost.
Labs	Pure-tone audiometry reveals sensorineural hearing loss; **discrimination of speech markedly reduced;** loudness recruitment absent; tone decay seen.
Imaging	CT: left **cerebellopontine-angle tumor** suggestive of acoustic neuroma.
Gross Pathology	**Encapsulated tumor** arising out of periphery of CN VIII (vestibular division) at cerebellopontine angle.
Micro Pathology	**Spindle cells** with tightly interlaced pattern (= ANTONI A) and **Verocay bodies.**
Treatment	Surgical resection curative.
Discussion	Tumors arise from the distal neurilemmal portion of the eighth nerve, usually from the vestibular division, and are correctly called schwannomas; they account for **80% of cerebellopontine tumors.** Tumors can be successfully removed, but cranial nerve palsies like CN VII nerve and deafness are common.

. . . .

SENSORINEURAL HEARING LOSS WITH ACOUSTIC NEUROMA

ID/CC	A 55-year-old male complains of progressively increasing **shortness of breath on exertion** for the past few months.
HPI	He also complains of nonproductive mild cough and has a **40-pack-year smoking history** but has no history of hemoptysis or occupational exposure to inorganic or organic dusts.
PE	VS: moderate tachypnea. PE: moderate respiratory distress, **using accessory muscles of respiration;** fullness of neck veins during expiration; chest **barrel shaped; percussion note hyperresonant; cardiac and liver dullness** are **obliterated;** scattered rhonchi bilaterally; **heart sounds heard distant** but normal.
Labs	ABGs: mild hypoxia with respiratory alkalosis. PFTs: increased residual volume; **decreased FEV_1/FVC ratio** (= OBSTRUCTIVE DISEASE PATTERN); decreased DL_{CO}.
Imaging	CXR (PA view): **hyperlucent** lung fields with a few **bullae;** flattening of diaphragm and elongated tubular heart shadow.
Gross Pathology	Air spaces dilated; **upper lobes most affected.**
Micro Pathology	Pattern of **centrilobular emphysema:** alveolar septa are visibly diminished in number along with increased air spaces.
Treatment	Cessation of smoking, bronchodilators, steroids in resistant cases, antibiotics during acute exacerbations, and home oxygen therapy.
Discussion	Emphysema is defined as abnormal permanent enlargement of the air spaces distal to the terminal bronchiole accompanied by the destruction of the alveolar walls; emphysema may involve the acinus and the lobule uniformly in a pattern called panacinar, or it may primarily involve the respiratory bronchioles, termed centriacinar. Panacinar emphysema is common in patients with **alpha-1-antitrypsin deficiency.** Centriacinar emphysema is commonly found in cigarette smokers and is rare in nonsmokers; it is usually more extensive and severe in the upper lobes.

. . . .

CHRONIC PULMONARY EMPHYSEMA

ID/CC A 50-year-old **farmer** presents with severe **shortness of breath** (= DYSPNEA) and **fatigue**.

HPI He also complains of a **dry cough** and **mild fever**. His symptoms are exacerbated when he works in the fields, especially when he comes into contact with **moldy hay**. He does not smoke and drinks alcohol occasionally.

PE VS: tachycardia; tachypnea; mild fever. PE: moderate respiratory distress; scattered rhonchi and **bilateral fine rales**.

Labs CBC: leukocytosis with shift to left. Elevated ESR; **serum antibodies against thermophilic *Actinomyces* organisms**; bronchoalveolar lavage shows marked lymphocytosis, primarily suppressor-cytotoxic T cells. PFTs: **restrictive lung disease** pattern.

Imaging CXR: bilateral **reticulonodular infiltrates with fibrosis**. CT: areas of ground-glass abnormalities with centrilobular peribronchial nodules.

Gross Pathology Fibrosis with honeycombing.

Micro Pathology Bronchoscopic lung biopsy reveals interstitial pneumonia with lymphocytes and plasma cells in alveolar walls as well as scattered focal granulomas with foreign body giant cells.

Treatment Strict avoidance of contact with aspergillus spores; steroids.

Discussion Hypersensitivity pneumonitis (allergic alveolitis) refers to interstitial lung disease that results from inhalation of organic antigens. Hypersensitivity pneumonitis is believed to have an immunologic basis (e.g., cytotoxic, immune complex, and cell-mediated reactions); **the most common form of hypersensitivity pneumonitis, called farmer's lung, is caused by inhalation of a thermophilic *Actinomyces* organism present in moldy hay and grain.** Other common causes of hypersensitivity pneumonitis include pigeon breeder's disease and bird fancier's disease, in which inhaled serum proteins from pigeons or parakeets induce the syndrome. Humidifier lung disease results from exposure to contaminated forced-air systems.

. . . .

HYPERSENSITIVITY PNEUMONITIS

ID/CC   A 65-year-old male complains of progressive shortness of breath on exertion.

HPI   The patient has **never smoked** cigarettes and has no history of exposure to occupational dusts or fumes; he has not had a productive cough or hemoptysis.

PE   VS: warm but **cyanosed;** tachycardia (HR 88); normotension. PE: **clubbing present;** JVP not elevated; heart sounds normal with no additional sounds or murmurs; respiratory examination reveals presence of bilateral **basal fine inspiratory crepitations.**

Labs   PFTs: **decreased DL_{CO};** desaturation with exercise; proportionately reduced FEV_1 and FVC so that ratio remained unchanged (due to restrictive disease). Bronchoalveolar lavage predominantly neutrophilic; serum calcium and ACE levels low.

Imaging CXR: reticulonodular shadows in both lower lung fields with occasional areas of **"honeycombing."** CT (high resolution): fibrosis in lower lung lobes suggestive of usual **interstitial pneumonitis pattern of IPF.**

Gross Pathology N/A

Micro Pathology Bronchoscopically obtained lung biopsy reveals presence of fibrosis, inflammatory round cell infiltrate, and thickening of the alveolar septa.

Treatment Systemic steroids.

Discussion The main differential diagnoses to consider are lung fibrosis associated with a connective tissue disorder (rule out by history and clinical exam), extrinsic alveolitis due to organic dusts, left-sided heart failure, sarcoidosis (rule out on basis of absence of any other system involvement, normal ACE levels, negative Kveim's test, and lack of hilar lymphadenopathy observed on CXR), lymphangitis carcinomatosa (rule out on biopsy and CT), and pneumoconiosis.

. . . .

IDIOPATHIC PULMONARY FIBROSIS (IPF)

ID/CC	A **28-year-old black female** complains of **fever, dyspnea, arthralgia, and erythematous, tender nodules** on both legs.
HPI	She has no history of foreign travel or contact with a tubercular patient.
PE	VS: fever. PE: tender, **erythematous nodules over extensor aspects of both legs** (= ERYTHEMA NODOSUM); arthralgias of both knees; splenomegaly.
Labs	CBC: **lymphopenia; eosinophilia.** Lytes: **elevated serum calcium; hypercalciuria. ACE levels elevated;** blood cultures negative; **Mantoux test negative;** fungal serology negative. PFTs: **evidence of restrictive changes.** Transbronchial lung biopsy ordered.
Imaging	CXR: **bilateral hilar lymphadenopathy** and right paratracheal adenopathy; **interstitial infiltrates;** no pleural effusion.
Gross Pathology	Firm nodules only a few millimeters in size in affected organs; can become confluent and give rise to larger nodules.
Micro Pathology	Lymph node biopsy reveals **noncaseating granulomas** with fibrotic acellular core surrounded by lymphocytes, epithelioid cells, and Langhans giant cells.
Treatment	**Corticosteroids.**
Discussion	May be asymptomatic; however, symptoms may be constitutional and involve many different organ systems, including the lungs, lymph nodes, skin, eye, upper respiratory tract, reticuloendothelial system, liver, kidney, nervous system, and heart. **FIRST AID** p.237

. . . .

SARCOIDOSIS

ID/CC	A 40-year-old male is brought to the ER with complaints of **sudden-onset, severe right-sided chest pain followed by severe difficulty in breathing.**
HPI	He is a chronic smoker and has predominantly **emphysematous** COPD.
PE	VS: severe tachycardia; tachypnea; hypotension; no fever. PE: **cyanosis; trachea shifted** to left; chest exam reveals **hyperresonant percussion note on right, diminished breath sounds,** and **decreased tactile fremitus.**
Labs	ABGs: hypoxemia. ECG: normal.
Imaging	CXR (after patient stabilizes): **right pneumothorax compressing lung parenchyma and shifting of mediastinum toward left.** Flattened left hemidiaphragm.
Gross Pathology	Pleural space is filled with air and lung is atelectatic (to demonstrate pneumothorax at autopsy, the chest cavity is opened underwater, letting air bubbles escape).
Micro Pathology	Section of lung shows collapsed alveolar spaces.
Treatment	Immediate life-saving treatment consists of inserting a wide-bore IV cannula on the affected side to decompress the pleural cavity if a chest drain is not immediately available; the wide-bore needle can then be replaced by a chest drain connected to an underwater seal.
Discussion	In tension pneumothorax, air enters the pleural space during inspiration and is prevented from escaping during expiration (because an airway or tissue flap acts as a one-way valve); there is a progressive increase in pleural air which is under pressure (i.e., tension). Tension pneumothorax occurs in only 1%–2% of cases of idiopathic spontaneous pneumothorax; it is a more common manifestation of the barotrauma that may occur during positive pressure mechanical ventilation.

TENSION PNEUMOTHORAX

ID/CC A 45-year-old **male** is seen with complaints of **sudden-onset, intense pain in his right big toe.**

HPI He had awakened in the middle of the night in pain, sweating profusely and shivering. His general practitioner two weeks ago prescribed a **thiazide diuretic** for mild to moderate hypertension.

PE VS: mild fever. PE: obese; in acute distress; right foot and ankle swollen; **marked redness and tenderness over metatarsophalangeal joint of big toe** that extends on to dorsum of foot.

Labs CBC: leukocytosis. Raised ESR; elevated serum uric acid; synovial fluid reveals **needle-shaped, negatively birefringent uric acid crystals.**

Imaging XR-Right Foot and Ankle: no specific abnormality in early phases (punched-out areas later).

Gross Pathology Acute attacks are characterized by signs of acute inflammation (chronic gout shows fibrosis of periarticular tissues and powdery, chalky-white deposits of **sodium urate crystals** called **tophi**).

Micro Pathology **PMNs and synovial proliferation in acute phase of gout** (in established lesions, needle-shaped crystals of urate salts are surrounded by foreign body giant cells, granulomas, and fibrosis).

Treatment Indomethacin or colchicine (less preferred due to GI side effects) for acute attacks; steroids for those with NSAID contraindications; avoid alcohol and diuretics (produces hyperuricemia) and lose weight; allopurinol (a xanthine oxidase inhibitor) in chronic phase to reduce uric acid production.

Discussion Gout is associated with hyperuricemia and deposition of urate crystals in joints, producing attacks of painful arthritis that may progress to chronic phase with **tophus** formation. Gout is seen predominantly in males (> 30 years), in postmenopausal females, and in children with leukemia or with HGPRTase deficiency (Lesch–Nyhan syndrome). **FIRST AID** p.237

ID/CC	A **2-year-old** white male child is seen with complaints of **fever** followed by a diffuse skin rash.
HPI	The child was apparently well a month ago, born to a couple after an uncomplicated pregnancy and delivery.
PE	VS: tachycardia; fever. PE: mild pallor; otoscopy of left ear reveals dull, poorly mobile tympanic membrane with pus behind it (= OTITIS MEDIA); generalized lymphadenopathy; hepatosplenomegaly; diffuse maculopapular eczematous rash.
Labs	CBC: anemia; thrombocytopenia with leukopenia (= PANCYTOPENIA); relative eosinophilia.
Imaging	CT-Abdomen: hepatosplenomegaly; XR: **cystic, rarefied lesions on skull and pelvis.**
Gross Pathology	Skin shows presence of extensive **eczematoid rash;** large destructive bone lesions found on skull and pelvis.
Micro Pathology	**Eosinophilic granulomatous lesions** in all involved organs; EM shows typical **Langerhans cells with characteristic Birbeck granules;** these cells were further found to be HLA-DR-positive and expressing **CD1 antigen.**
Treatment	Corticosteroids; surgery or radiotherapy for localized bone disease.
Discussion	Letterer–Siwe is an acute or subacute clinical syndrome of unknown etiology affecting children less than three years old. It is marked by fever due to localized infection, followed by a diffuse maculopapular eczematous purpuric skin rash and subsequent hepatosplenomegaly and generalized lymphadenopathy. It shows similarities to acute leukemia and other infectious processes. Diabetes insipidus, exophthalmos, and bone lesions are usually seen in combination.

. . . .

LETTERER–SIWE DISEASE

ID/CC   A **60-year-old obese female** is seen with complaints of gradually progressing **stiffness and pain after use of the right knee.**

HPI   The pain and stiffness are accompanied by swelling and deformity of the joint. She also reports difficulty walking and limitation of movement.

PE   Tenderness, pain, and crepitus of right knee on motion; firm swelling (caused by underlying bony proliferations) and joint effusion; fixed deformities: bony enlargement and a varus angulation, causing limited motion at joint; hands show **bony swellings on distal interphalangeal joints** (= HEBERDEN'S NODES).

Labs   Synovial fluid shows no evidence of inflammation; normal viscosity and mucin clot tests; protein, glucose, and complement levels also normal; serum rheumatoid factor not raised.

Imaging   XR-Right Knee (AP and lateral views): narrowing of joint space (medial > lateral); subchondral bone sclerosis; subchondral cysts and osteophytes.

Gross Pathology   Late stages of the disease show **eburnation** of joint surface, **remodeling** of joint surface, **osteophytes** around lateral margins of joint, subchondral bone cysts, and bone sclerosis.

Micro Pathology   Loss of articular cartilage, bone resorption, and irregular and variable new bone and cartilage formation.

Treatment   Pain relief, improvement of mobility, and correction of deformity; joint replacement.

Discussion   A condition affecting the large weight-bearing joints, osteoarthritis is characterized by the degeneration of articular cartilage and progressive destruction and remodeling of the joint structures. It is more common in women, and its incidence increases with age, particularly after 55.
FIRST AID p.236

. . . .

OSTEOARTHRITIS

ID/CC	An **18-year-old male** presents with a **fracture of the shaft of the femur following a minor fall.**
HPI	He also complains of **facial asymmetry,** deviation of the angle of the mouth, drooling of saliva, and inability to whistle. **His father suffers from a bone disease.**
PE	Fracture of shaft of left femur; right facial nerve palsy, lower motor neuron type (entrapment neuropathy).
Labs	**Serum acid phosphatase and creatine kinase (brain isozyme) increased;** serum PTH increased; serum calcium and calcitriol normal.
Imaging	XR: **generalized symmetric osteosclerosis; "Erlenmeyer flask" deformity** of distal left femur in addition to fracture of shaft; alternating dense and lucent bands seen in metaphyses; cranium thickened and dense; paranasal and nasal sinuses underpneumatized; vertebrae show, on lateral view, **"bone in bone"** appearance.
Gross Pathology	N/A
Micro Pathology	Histopathologic studies reveal profound **deficiency of osteoclast function** and **primary spongiosa** (calcified cartilage deposited during endochondral bone formation) occurring away from growth plate (characteristic histologic finding of osteopetrosis).
Treatment	Steroid therapy with low-calcium, high-phosphate diet; management of fracture and surgical decompression of facial nerve.
Discussion	A **defect in bone resorption** secondary to **impaired osteoclast action** is the key factor in the pathogenesis of the disease.

OSTEOPETROSIS

ID/CC	A **60-year-old woman** visits her physician complaining of severe low back pain after a fall from her bed.
HPI	Onset of **menopause** was at 48 years. The patient is **not receiving hormone replacement therapy;** she suffered a Colles' fracture last year that is malunited. Directed history reveals **loss of height and a mild hunchback deformity.**
PE	Patient thin; kyphosis noted; percussion over dorsolumbar spine exquisitely tender; right wrist: malunited Colles' fracture.
Labs	Serum calcium, phosphates and alkaline phosphatase and PTH within normal limits; **densitometry** used to quantify osteoporosis.
Imaging	XR-Dorsolumbar Spine: loss of vertical height of L4 vertebra (due to collapse and compression fracture) and kyphosis. DEXA (dual energy X-ray absorptiometry): reduced bone mass.
Gross Pathology	**Thin cortex; thin trabeculae, reduced in number,** resulting in increased medullary space; obvious fracture with healing and deformity; **collapse of vertebral bodies** with kyphoscoliosis.
Micro Pathology	Bone biopsy: thin but normally formed cortex and trabeculae; normal calcification; trabeculae very slender; microfractures and fracture healing may be evident.
Treatment	High-protein diet; **calcium supplementation; androgens** (anabolic effect on bone matrix); **estrogens** (shown to halt progressive bone loss); **vitamin D; exercise** (weight bearing acts as stimulus to bone formation); bracing of spine to prevent further fractures and deformity in a severely osteoporotic spine.
Discussion	Osteoporosis is characterized by a **reduction of total skeletal mass due to increased bone resorption** (bone formation is normal); there is greater loss of trabecular than compact bone; it results in a predisposition to pathologic fracture. **FIRST AID** p.242

. . . .

OSTEOPOROSIS

ID/CC	A 70-year-old female is seen with complaints of **inability to comb her hair, put on her coat, and get up from her chair for the past six months.**
HPI	She complains of **shoulder and pelvic area stiffness** and pain (especially during **morning hours**), fever, malaise, and fatigue.
PE	VS: low-grade fever. PE: pallor; stiff, deliberate movements; affected joints show restricted movement; muscle strength normal; remainder of physical exam normal.
Labs	CBC: normochromic anemia. **ESR markedly elevated;** other acute-phase reactants such as fibrinogen and alpha-2-globulin levels increased.
Imaging	XR: normal.
Gross Pathology	N/A
Micro Pathology	N/A
Treatment	Low-dose oral steroids; watch for development of giant cell arteritis, which threatens vision in up to one-third of patients.
Discussion	Polymyalgia rheumatica is characterized by **aching and morning stiffness** in the shoulder and hip girdles, the proximal extremities, the neck, and the torso; the spectrum of disease includes giant cell arteritis. Mean age at onset is 70; women are affected twice as often as men. A strong association with **HLA-DR4** has been observed. Some cases recur and some patients become steroid dependent.

· ·

POLYMYALGIA RHEUMATICA

ID/CC	A 60-year-old woman presents with **swelling and pain** in the left **knee after undergoing a major surgical procedure**.
HPI	She has no history of fever or trauma.
PE	Left knee warm and crepitant upon movement, which is restricted and painful; positive patellar tap indicates an effusion.
Labs	Synovial fluid from left knee shows increased leukocyte count, predominantly neutrophils; normal uric acid levels; **birefringent crystals**, both free and within leukocytes; crystals show a **weakly positive birefringence and are rhomboid in shape**.
Imaging	XR-Left Knee: punctate and **linear calcification in articular cartilage** (= CHONDROCALCINOSIS).
Gross Pathology	N/A
Micro Pathology	N/A
Treatment	**Anti-inflammatory drugs**, including salicylates, phenylbutazone, indomethacin, and glucocorticoids, are effective to varying degrees; joint aspiration may help; triamcinolone intra-articularly for resistant cases.
Discussion	The term "pseudogout" refers to acute attacks of arthritis associated with the presence in the synovial fluid of birefringent crystals, both free and within leukocytes. **Pseudogout crystals show a weakly positive birefringence, whereas monosodium urate crystals show a strongly negative birefringence.** Generally, pseudogout crystals are also stubbier and more rhomboid than urate crystals. Radiographic evidence of calcinosis (presumably CPPD crystals) in cartilage and other structures is often present. The typical pattern involves calcification in articular cartilage, fibrocartilage (meniscus of the knee, pubic symphysis, anulus fibrosus), synovium, fibrous capsules, tendons, and bursae. **FIRST AID** p.237

. . . .

PSEUDOGOUT

ID/CC	A **30-year-old** white **female** complains that the **fingers** of both hands **become pale** on **exposure to cold.**
HPI	At times, the pain is also precipitated by **emotional stress.** She is not taking any drugs and does not suffer from any other diagnosed ailment (e.g., collagen vascular disease; thyroid, adrenal, or pituitary diseases).
PE	Peripheral pulses palpable; **dipping patient's hands in cold water precipitated pain and resulted in development of digital blanching;** rewarming caused cyanosis and rubor of fingers.
Labs	Laboratory tests exclude all causes of secondary Raynaud's disease (collagen vascular diseases and blood dyscrasias).
Imaging	N/A
Gross Pathology	N/A
Micro Pathology	N/A
Treatment	Protect hands and feet from exposure to cold; drug therapy with a calcium channel blocker such as nifedipine or a sympatholytic agent such as reserpine or guanethidine.
Discussion	Primary Raynaud's phenomenon, or Raynaud's disease, is a vasospastic disorder, whereas secondary Raynaud's phenomenon occurs as a complication of systemic disease; scleroderma, systemic lupus erythematosus, and related immunologic disorders. Women are affected approximately five times more than men, and the age at presentation is usually between 30 and 40 years. The fingers are involved more frequently than the toes.

ID/CC	A **5-year-old male** is brought to a physician with sudden-onset progressive severe **pain, swelling, and redness** of the right knee joint.
HPI	He has had a **high-grade fever** for the past two days. A few days ago he **injured his right leg, and the injury subsequently became infected;** he is now unable to move his right leg properly.
PE	VS: fever. PE: infected wound on right leg; right **knee red, swollen, and tender;** all movements restricted by pain.
Labs	CBC: **neutrophilic leukocytosis** with shift to the left. Elevated ESR; **synovial fluid (obtained following joint aspiration) opaque and yellowish;** Gram stain reveals **gram-positive cocci in clusters;** culture yields coagulase-positive *S. aureus.*
Imaging	XR-Right Knee: early, soft tissue swelling and joint effusion; late, articular erosions and reactive sclerosis. NUC-Gallium Scan: increased uptake by right knee joint.
Gross Pathology	N/A
Micro Pathology	N/A
Treatment	**Broad-spectrum parenteral antibiotics** initially, then specific antibiotics following culture sensitivity reports; if necessary, joint may be opened, washed, and closed with a suction drain and immobilized until signs of inflammation subside.
Discussion	Caused by pyogenic organisms and more common among children, especially males. *S. aureus* is the most common cause; other organisms include streptococci, gonococci, pneumococci, and *N. meningitides.* Organisms reach the joint via hematogenous routes (most common; primary focus may be a pyoderma, throat infection, etc.), secondary to adjacent osteomyelitis, or via penetrating wounds, or may be iatrogenic.

· ·

SEPTIC ARTHRITIS

ID/CC	A 65-year-old male presents with **acute urinary retention.**
HPI	For the past few years, he has noted an **increased frequency** of micturition along with increased **hesitancy, urgency,** decreased force and stream of urine, and a feeling of **incomplete evacuation** of the bladder. For the past few months he has begun to experience **increasing fatigability and lassitude.**
PE	Patient is anemic; bladder full on abdominal examination; rectal exam reveals **grade III prostate enlargement along with firm, non-nodular, and mobile mass overlying rectal mucosa;** after catheterization, abdominal examination reveals bilateral **masses** in lumbar regions.
Labs	Lytes: hypocalcemia; hyperphosphatemia. **Elevated BUN and creatinine.** UA: proteinuria; **no RBCs or casts seen.**
Imaging	US-Kidneys: **bilateral hydroureter and hydronephrosis.**
Gross Pathology	N/A
Micro Pathology	In addition to hydronephrosis and hydroureter, interstitial kidney disease is seen on microscopic examination.
Treatment	**Transurethral resection** of the prostate (TURP) to relieve the obstruction is the basic and most useful step.
Discussion	Obstructive nephropathy results from the **impaired outflow of urine** but may also **produce chronic interstitial damage.** Obstructive nephropathy from congenital abnormalities is common in childhood and in individuals older than 60 years, when benign prostatic hypertrophy and prostatic and gynecologic cancers become more common.

· ·

BLADDER OUTLET OBSTRUCTION, REFLUX NEPHROPATHY

ID/CC	A 45-year-old **black** male presents with uncontrolled **hypertension** and complains of severe occipital headache and ringing in his ears.
HPI	He also reports **markedly diminished urine output over the past 24 hours.** On directed questioning, he also reports **some visual blurring.**
PE	VS: **severe hypertension.** PE: funduscopy reveals presence of **papilledema** with hypertensive **retinopathy.**
Labs	UA: proteinuria; microscopic hematuria; **red cell casts. Elevated BUN and creatinine.** CBC: microangiopathic hemolytic anemia. ECG: left-axis deviation with left ventricular hypertrophy.
Imaging	Echo: concentric left ventricular hypertrophy with reduced ejection fraction. US-Abdomen: presence of **parenchymal renal disease in normal-sized kidneys** (unlike that of benign nephrosclerosis, where there are bilateral contracted kidneys).
Gross Pathology	N/A
Micro Pathology	Pathologic changes include **fibrinoid necrosis of arterioles** (= NECROTIZING ARTERIOLITIS), **hyperplastic arteriolosclerosis** (= "ONION SKINNING"), and necrotizing glomerulitis associated with a thrombotic microangiopathy.
Treatment	**Reduction of diastolic blood pressure to at least 100 mmHg, and to maintain urine output > 20 mL/hour.**
Discussion	**Sodium nitroprusside** is the safest and most effective drug for use in hypertensive emergencies; because it does not impair myocardial blood flow, it is especially useful in underlying ischemic heart disease. However, it is metabolized to cyanide and thiocyanate; therefore, prolonged use may lead to cyanide toxicity or to thiocyanate toxicity. Blood thiocyanate levels should be determined frequently.

. . . .

HYPERTENSIVE RENAL DISEASE

ID/CC	A **30-year-old black woman** presents with **pain** in both her knee **joints** and in the small joints of the hand together with mild fever, anorexia, weight loss, and loss of hair.
HPI	She also has a history of **recurrent oral ulcerations** and a **photosensitive skin rash**. No joint deformities are reported.
PE	VS: **hypertension**. PE: oral **aphthous ulcers** noted; erythematous **photosensitive skin rash;** "**butterfly rash**" over malar area of face; pallor; no abdominal or renal bruits heard.
Labs	CBC: normocytic, normochromic **anemia.** UA: microscopic hematuria with **RBC casts** in addition to proteinuria. **Elevated BUN and creatinine; antinuclear antibodies positive** in high titer; LE cell phenomenon positive; **anti-Sm antibody and anti-ds DNA antibody positive;** VDRL **positive** but FTA-ABS negative.
Imaging	N/A
Gross Pathology	N/A
Micro Pathology	Renal biopsy reveals features of **diffuse proliferative glomerulonephritis.** Electron microscopy reveals **immune complex deposits** that are typically **subendothelial** and form "**wire loops.**"
Treatment	Corticosteroids; cytotoxic drugs (cyclophosphamide, azathioprine and chlorambucil); long-term hemodialysis or transplant.
Discussion	There are five patterns of lupus nephritis. Class I is normal by light, EM, and immunofluorescence microscopy. Class II presents as **mesangial lupus glomerulonephritis** and is found in about 25% of patients; it is associated with minimal hematuria or proteinuria. Class III is characterized by **focal proliferative** glomerulonephritis and is associated with recurrent hematuria and mild renal insufficiency. Class IV is described in this case and is by far the most common form. Class V presents as **membranous glomerulonephritis** and is seen in 15% of cases; it induces severe proteinuria or nephrotic syndrome. **FIRST AID** p.237

· ·

LUPUS NEPHRITIS

ID/CC	A newborn baby is evaluated for **ambiguous external genitalia.**
HPI	The baby was delivered vaginally at full term without any pre-, intra-, or postnatal complications; the mother did not take **hormones** or any other **drugs during pregnancy.**
PE	Incompletely virilized external genitalia; hypospadias; **bilateral inguinal swelling.**
Labs	Karyotype: 46 XY. Müllerian structures absent; inguinal swellings proved to be **maldescended dysgenetic testes.**
Imaging	US: absence of müllerian structures and presence of dysgenic testes.
Gross Pathology	N/A
Micro Pathology	Testes characterized by **seminiferous tubule degeneration** and invasion by connective tissue arranged in whorls.
Treatment	**Gonadectomy** to protect against increased risk of testicular tumor; **hormone replacement** therapy.
Discussion	The incidence of **gonadal tumors in dysgenetic gonads** may reach up to 30%, making orchiectomy and subsequent hormone replacement the best therapeutic option.

ID/CC	A 45-year-old man with a high-grade **non-Hodgkin's lymphoma** develops **oliguria, severe malaise, and fatigue** 36 hours following **chemotherapy treatment.**
HPI	N/A
PE	Carpopedal **spasm** present; neither kidney is palpable; urinary bladder is empty.
Labs	Lytes: hyperkalemia, **hyperuricemia,** and hyperphosphatemia with secondary hypocalcemia. **BUN and creatinine and elevated.** UA: acidic urine with numerous **needle-shaped crystals;** no casts or cells seen.
Imaging	N/A
Gross Pathology	N/A
Micro Pathology	N/A
Treatment	Maintenance of good hydration, brisk diuresis and **pretreatment with allopurinol** are keys to prevention of this syndrome; once acute renal failure has developed, fluid and electrolyte balance must be maintained and dialysis may be necessary.
Discussion	Tumor lysis syndrome is most often seen in patients with **lymphoma or leukemia** but is also seen in patients with a variety of solid tumors. The presence of **a large tumor burden, a high growth fraction, an increased pretreatment LDH level and uric acid level,** or preexisting renal insufficiency increases the likelihood that a patient will develop tumer lysis syndrome. Increased levels of uric acid, xanthine, and phosphate may result in precipitation of these substances in the kidney. Renal sludging and acute renal insufficiency or failure further aggravate the metabolic abnormality.

· ·

URATE NEPHROPATHY

From the authors of *Underground Clinical Vignettes*

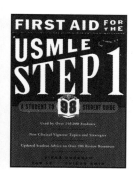

A true classic used by over 200,000 students around the world. The '99 edition features details on the new computerized test, new color plates and thoroughly updated high-yield facts and book reviews. Bi-directional links with the *Underground Clinical Vignettes Step 1* series. ISBN 0-8385-2612-8.

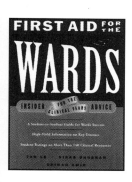

This high-yield student-to-student guide is designed to help students make the transition from the basic sciences to the hospital wards and succeed on their clinical rotations. The book features an orientation to the hospital environment, tips on being an effective and efficient junior medical student, student-proven advice tailored to each core rotation, a database of high-yield clinical facts, and recommendations for clinical pocket books, texts, and references. ISBN 0-8385-2595-4.

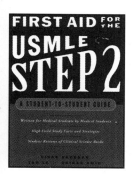

This entirely rewritten second edition now follows in the footsteps of *First Aid for the USMLE Step 1*. Features an exam preparation guide geared to the new computerized test, basic science and clinical high-yield facts, color plates and ratings of USMLE Step 2 books and software. Bi-directional links with the *Underground Clinical Vignettes Step 2* series.

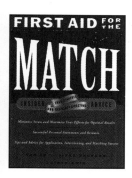

This top rated (5 stars, *Doody Review*) student-to-student guide helps medical students effectively and efficiently navigate the residency application process, helping them make the most of their limited time, money, and energy. The book draws on the advice and experiences of successful student applicants as well as residency directors. Also featured are application and interview tips tailored to each specialty, successful personal statements and CVs with analyses, current trends, and common interview questions with suggested strategies for responding. ISBN 0-8385-2596-2.

The *First Aid* series by Appleton & Lange...the review book leader.
Available through your local health sciences bookstore !

About the Authors

. . . .

VIKAS BHUSHAN, MD

Vikas is a diagnostic radiologist in Los Angeles and the series editor for *Underground Clinical Vignettes*. His interests include traveling, reading, writing, and world music. He is single and can be reached at vbhushan@aol.com

CHIRAG AMIN, MD

Chirag is an orthopedics resident at Orlando Regional Medical Center. He plans on pursuing a spine fellowship. He can be reached at chiragamin@aol.com

TAO LE, MD

Tao is completing a medicine residency at Yale-New Haven Hospital and is applying for a fellowship in allergy and immunology. He is married to Thao, who is a pediatrics resident. He can be reached at taotle@aol.com

HOANG NGUYEN

Hoang (Henry) is a third-year medical student at Northwestern University. Henry is single and lives in Chicago, where he spends his free time writing, reading, and enjoying music. He can be reached at hbnguyen@nwu.edu

ASHRAF ZAMAN

Ashraf trained in Internal Medicine in New Delhi, India and hopes to begin a residency in the US in 1999. He is recently engaged to be married and lives in Michigan. He can be reached at fauziyah@aol.com